THE HEALING POWER
OF MINDFULNESS

MEDITATION IS NOT WHAT YOU THINK: Mindfulness and Why It Is So Important
FALLING AWAKE: How to Practice Mindfulness in Everyday Life
MINDFULNESS FOR ALL: The Wisdom to Transform the World

MINDFULNESS:
Diverse Perspectives on Its Meaning, Origins, and Applications
(editor, with J. Mark G. Williams)

MINDFULNESS FOR BEGINNERS:
Reclaiming the Present Moment—and Your Life

THE MIND'S OWN PHYSICIAN:
A Scientific Dialogue with the Dalai Lama on the Healing Power of Meditation
(editor, with Richard J. Davidson)

LETTING EVERYTHING BECOME YOUR TEACHER:
100 Lessons in Mindfulness

ARRIVING AT YOUR OWN DOOR:
108 Lessons in Mindfulness

THE MINDFUL WAY THROUGH DEPRESSION:
Freeing Yourself from Chronic Unhappiness
(with Mark Williams, John Teasdale, and Zindel Segal)

COMING TO OUR SENSES:
Healing Ourselves and the World Through Mindfulness

EVERYDAY BLESSINGS:
The Inner Work of Mindful Parenting
(with Myla Kabat-Zinn)

WHEREVER YOU GO, THERE YOU ARE:
Mindfulness Meditation in Everyday Life

FULL CATASTROPHE LIVING:
Using the Wisdom of Your Body and Mind to Face Stress, Pain, and Illness

THE HEALING POWER
OF MINDFULNESS

A New Way of Being

JON KABAT-ZINN

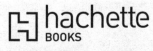

BOOKS

NEW YORK   BOSTON

Hachette Books
Hachette Book Group
1290 Avenue of the Americas
New York, NY 10104
hachettebooks.com
twitter.com/hachettebooks

Originally published in hardcover as part of *Coming to Our Senses* by Hyperion in January 2005.

First Edition: November 2018

Credits and permissions appear beginning on p. 225 and constitute a continuation of the copyright page.

Hachette Books is a division of Hachette Book Group, Inc.
The Hachette Books name and logo are trademarks of Hachette Book Group, Inc.

The publisher is not responsible for websites (or their content) that are not owned by the publisher.

The Hachette Speakers Bureau provides a wide range of authors for speaking events. To find out more, go to www.hachettespeakersbureau.com or call (866) 376-6591.

Library of Congress Control Number: 2018943583

ISBNs: 978-0-316-41176-9 (trade paperback), 978-0-316-52205-2 (ebook)

Printed in the United States of America

LSC-H

10 9 8 7 6 5 4 3 2 1

for Myla
for Tayo, Stella, Asa, and Toby
for Will and Teresa
for Naushon
for Serena
for the memory of Sally and Elvin
and Howie and Roz

for all those who care

for what is possible

for what is so

for wisdom

for clarity

for kindness

for love

CONTENTS

FOREWORD

Mindfulness is a wise and potentially healing way of being in relationship to what befalls us in life. And, improbable as it may sound, that includes anything and everything you or any of us might encounter. Even when facing extremely challenging life circumstances or in their aftermath, there is profound promise associated with the cultivation of mindfulness. You may be surprised at just how wide-ranging its effects are or could be if you are open to at least putting your toe in the waters of formal and informal meditation practice and seeing what unfolds.

As the majority of people who take the MBSR (mindfulness-based stress reduction) program discover, as well as those who come to mindfulness through some other door, the curriculum is none other than life itself: facing and embracing your life as it is, including whatever you may be dealing with in any given moment. And underscore *"whatever."* The challenge, as it always is with mindfulness as a practice and as a way of being, is this: How are you going to be in wise relationship to this moment as it is, however it is, including all the annoying, unwanted, and terrifying elements that arise on occasion and need facing? Is it possible to be open to the lessons you can learn from approaching life—and all your moments—in a radical new way?

In my vocabulary, the word *healing* is best described as coming to terms with things as they are. It doesn't mean fixing, and it doesn't mean curing, as in fully restoring an original condition, or making whatever it is that is problematic simply go away.

The process and practice of coming to terms with things as they are very much does mean investigating for yourself whether you actually even know how things are or if you just think you do—and therefore, in the very way you choose to go about thinking about your situation, mis-take the actuality of things for your narratives about them. Coming to terms with things as they are involves experimenting with how you, we, all of us might redefine and thereby transform our relationship with what is actually so, including our obvious not knowing of how things are going to unfold even in the very next moment. This inward stance opens up boundless possibilities we could never have conceived of. Why? Because our very thinking patterns are so limiting, weighed down as they are by our astonishingly unexamined habits of mind. In this book we are going to be cracking those habits wide open, over and over again, virtually moment by moment, thereby apprehending the openings and opportunities that arise when we do so; when, in Derek Walcott's words, you "greet yourself arriving at your own door."

*

In my travels, I frequently encounter people who tell me, unbidden, that mindfulness has given their life back to them. They often share their stories of unbelievably horrendous life circumstances, events, or diagnoses that nobody would ever wish on anybody. That is the way they usually phrase it: "Mindfulness (or "the practice") has given my life back to me," or "has saved my life." It is frequently accompanied by an outpouring of gratitude. When this sentiment is communicated to me either face to face or in a letter or an e-mail, it invariably sounds so authentic and unique that I have the definite sense that it is not being exaggerated.

Interestingly, every single person who engages in the practice of mindfulness fairly systematically over time has followed her or his or their own unique trajectory while at the same time, using the same invariant set of formal meditation practices that we use in MBSR (the body scan, sitting meditation, mindful yoga, and mindful walking) as described in Book 2 of this series, *Falling Awake*, as well as, of course, by bringing mindfulness into their everyday encounters with life in whatever ways they can manage, always unique.

Here is an expression of such gratitude that I received recently in an e-mail passed on by my publisher in the UK, to which the writer had given the subject line "A Word of Appreciation":

Dear Professor Kabat-Zinn

Having read all your books (some more than once) and survived what was described as terminal esophageal cancer, I write to let you know how important a part they played in my recovery. It's now five years since the day I was (rather heartlessly) told in July "You might last till Christmas. Some last longer. If you need anything, just call the hospice."

The chronology of my journey is fraught with mistakes, including the use of the wrong patient notes when planning radical chemo and radiotherapy. Two vertebrae in my spine were broken as a result of the radiotherapy overdose, but here I am on 19th October 2017 into the first six weeks of an MSc in Mindfulness at Aberdeen University. The dream is to be fully qualified to help seriously ill patients in our local cancer support centres using techniques I learned from your CDs, videos, and books. Only fully qualified volunteers are allowed to work with patients.

Your Full Catastrophe Living *inspired me and became my bible during my lowest phase along with* Wherever You Go, There You Are. *At the moment I'm planning the first major 8,000 word essay on this degree course and am told that my theme ('Meditation Heals') is not ideal for academic research. I find this puzzling and wonder if you could advise me on where I should be looking for inspiration…*

It is no exaggeration to say that my readings of your work have saved my life and I'm making the most of every breath I was told I wouldn't be taking. I would greatly appreciate a word of guidance from you as I attempt to realize this dream of effectively helping sick patients discover their own power to heal themselves. How best can this become an academic study?

> WITH GRATITUDE AND WARM
> GREETINGS FROM ABERDEEN
>
> MARGARET DONALD
> *P.S.: I'm going to be 80 next year so every minute counts!*

Of course I wrote back. And among other things, I suggested to Margaret that she was so much more aligned with where academic medicine is heading than her advisors seem to be from their comment about academic research. I gave her a number of references to studies in the scientific literature supporting her choice of thesis topic and that use words such as "meditation" and "healing" in tandem.

*

When volunteers in various studies are put into brain scanners and told to do nothing, to just lie there, it turns out a major network in a diffuse region of the cerebral cortex located underneath the midline of the forehead and extending back becomes exceedingly active. This network, comprised of a number of different specialized structures, has come to be known as the *default mode network* (DMN) because what happens when we are told to "do nothing" and "just lie there" in the scanner is that we *default* to mind wandering. And guess where a lot of the mind-wandering carries us? You guessed it... to musing about our favorite subject—me of course! We fall into narratives about the past (my past), the future (my future), emotions (my worries, my anger, my depression), various life circumstances (my stress, my pressure, my successes, my failures, what is wrong with the country, with the world, with "them"). ... You get the idea.

Interestingly enough, when people are trained in MBSR for eight weeks, one study—conducted at the University of Toronto*—showed that after the program, activity in the DMN decreased while another more lateral (on the side of the head) brain network became more active as the study subjects lay in the scanner. This second network has been termed the *experiential network*. When asked about their experiences in the scanner, subjects who had been through the eight weeks of training in MBSR reported that they were just there, just breathing, simply aware of their body, their thoughts, their feelings, sounds, as they were lying there.

So perhaps, at least metaphorically (a lot more research would need to be conducted to say for sure) mindfulness practice leads to shifting the default mode from unaware (we could say *mindless*) self-preoccupation, mind wandering, narrative building, and being lost in thought, to being more present, more mindful, more aware, even as thinking and emotions continue of course to bubble up.

This study showed that the two networks (narrative vs experiential) become uncoupled after eight weeks of MBSR. Both networks continue to function, of course. After all, it is important for creativity and the imagination to daydream at times.† It is also very important to differentiate your past from your present from your imagined future, as the story about my father in the chapter "Orienting in Time and Space" will show. But after eight weeks of practicing mindfulness, it may be that the experiential, outside-of-time lateral network in the cortex somehow modulates the midline DMN so that, together, there might be greater wisdom and freedom of choice available in any

---

* Farb et al, 2007. Attending to the present: mindfulness meditation reveals distinct neural modes of self-reference. Social Cognitive and Affective Neuroscience Advance Access published August 13, 2007

† Mind-wandering and daydreaming are defined differently. Mind-wandering occurs during particular tasks, such as reading or meditation, when you are trying to stay focused. Daydreaming, as defined, happens at times when you are not trying to stay focused to accomplish a task. See Amishi Jha: https://www.youtube.com/watch?v=14gwYLg19zo ~ 33 minutes; see also "How to train your wandering mind": https://www.ted.com/talks/amishi_jha_how_to_tame_your_wandering_mind/transcript.

moment, rather than mere automaticity and habitual belief in tacit narratives of a self that is far too small to come close to who and what you actually are in your fullness, right here, right now.

*

In the thirteen years since *Coming to Our Senses* first came out, the science of mindfulness and the evidence for its clinical effectiveness have exploded. Among the findings are changes in the size and thickness of various brain structures in people practicing mindfulness, as well as increased functional connectivity between many different regions of the brain. There are studies showing changes in gene expression at the level of our chromosomes—what are called "epigenetic effects"—as well studies showing effects on telomere length, a biological measure of the impact of the stress in our lives, especially when it is severe. The cumulative thrust of the evidence from such studies and hundreds more appearing each year point to there being something about the practice of mindfulness that can have a major impact on our biology, our psychology, and even on the ways we interact with each other, our social psychology. While scientific research on meditation is still in its infancy, it is much more mature than it was in 2005. If you are interested in some of the most robust findings, many of which come, on the one hand, from studying monastics with tens of thousands of lifetime hours of meditation practice, but also from studies of people going through training in MBSR and MBCT, I suggest you take a look at the book *Altered Traits* by my colleagues Richard Davidson and Daniel Goleman, which came out in October of 2017. It summarizes many of the best and most well-designed studies and their outcomes. Because the field is now so extensive and growing so rapidly, I have not described more recent studies in detail in this book, although some are mentioned in passing in the text. A range of excellent recent books on the subject, mainly written by the scientists themselves for a lay readership are listed in the Related Reading section of this volume, along with some edited volumes that are targeted to a more professional scientific and medical audience, if you want to explore the cutting edge of this rapidly growing field for yourself.

*

When we extend the formal meditation practice into everyday living, life itself becomes our best mindfulness teacher. It also provides the perfect curriculum for healing, starting from exactly where you already are. The prognosis is excellent: that you too can benefit from this new way of being if you throw yourself wholeheartedly into the practice and make use of the various doorways available to you by virtue of who you are and the circumstances in which you find yourself. Every circumstance, however unwanted or painful, is potentially a door into healing. In the world of mindfulness as a practice and as a way of being, there are many, many doors. All lead into the very same room, the room of awareness itself, the room of your own heart, the room of your own intrinsic wholeness and beauty. And both that wholeness and that beauty are already here, and already yours, along with your intrinsic capacity for wakefulness, and thus, wisdom, even under the most trying circumstances.

Taking up the regular practice of mindfulness involves a major lifestyle change, as the participants in MBSR soon discover for themselves, although they are always told about it before they enroll. But when we do take on the rigorous discipline of a daily formal mindfulness practice as an experiment, and we engage in it as wholeheartedly as we can manage on any given day, we soon discover that we have a lot of degrees of freedom in how we choose to be in relationship with the unwanted or the frightening in our life without denying how unwanted and how frightening things may be. Within the very cultivation of mindfulness itself, as a formal meditation practice and as a way of being, we discover that we have powerful innate resources that we can draw upon in the face of what is unwanted, stressful, painful, or terrifying. We learn that we have countless opportunities to *turn toward* and to *befriend* whatever arises rather than to run away from it all or wall it off—to put out the welcome mat so to speak. Why? For the simple reason that it is already here. And the same applies to the wanted, the pleasant, the seductive, to entanglements of all kinds. Those experiences too can become objects of our attention so that we can perhaps be less caught by them or even addicted to them in ways that cause us and others harm or deflect us from our larger intentions and purpose.

This is precisely where mindfulness comes in. It is indeed a new way of being...a new way of *being in relationship to things as they are in this moment*, whether or not we like the circumstances we find ourselves in, and no matter what we think might be the implications those circumstances could portend for the future. In key moments, through the practice itself, we can explore and learn to abide in not knowing, and having that not knowing be OK, at least for now. Getting more familiar and even comfortable with knowing that we don't know is its own form of profound and healing intelligence. For one thing, it frees us from extremely limiting or largely inaccurate narratives, often fear-based, which we never tire of telling ourselves but hardly ever examine as to whether they are actually true, or true enough for the circumstances we find ourselves in. Most thoughts that have the word *should* in them probably fall into this category. We think things should be a certain way, but is that actually true?

This new way of being invites what might at first seem to be a tiny shift in how you see yourself and how you see the world. However tiny it may be, it is also huge, profound, and possibly liberating, as it was for Margaret Donald, who wrote the above letter. When people speak, often with great emotion, of the practice giving their life back to them or saving their life, this tiny shift, which is not so tiny, into a new way of being is what I suspect they are referring to.

With ongoing tending, with tenderness, with nurturing—which is what the formal and informal mindfulness practices that are described in detail in the second book in this series, *Falling Awake*, are all about— we are now in a position to enter into and adopt mindfulness as a way of being. If mindfulness were a multifaceted diamond, each chapter might be thought of as one of a potentially infinite number of unique facets of that diamond, each a gateway into the crystal lattice structure of your own wholeness and your beauty, just as you are in this present moment.

Or, switching and mixing metaphors, we could say that mindfulness offers us a set of finely crafted lenses through which we can glimpse different ways of looking deeply into whatever arises in our life—wanted or unwanted—afresh in each moment, putting out the welcome mat for it all. In Part 2, I offer a broad range of such lenses and circumstances, many from my own experience. But there are an infinite number that will flow from your own life and your own cultivation of mindfulness if you engage in it wholeheartedly, just as an experiment for a time to see for yourself what might unfold.

Ultimately, through one or more of these lenses, perhaps you will come to use your own unique life circumstances and challenges to, as suggested in the last chapter of this book, greet yourself arriving at your own door, and thus recognize, recover, and embody your own original fullness and beauty. This can only unfold moment by moment, especially if you choose to live your life as if it really mattered in the only moment you or any of us will ever have.

As we often remind people in the hospital who come to the Stress Reduction Clinic for training in MBSR, "as long as you are breathing, there is more right with you than wrong with you, no matter what is wrong." Cultivating mindfulness is a way to pour energy in the form of attention, awareness, and acceptance into what is already right with you, what is already whole, as a complement to, not a substitute for, whatever help and support and treatments you may be receiving or need—if you need any at all—and see what happens.

I wish you all the best in this adventure of a lifetime.

Jon Kabat-Zinn
Northampton, MA
May 16, 2018

PART 1

HEALING POSSIBILITIES

The Realm of Mind and Body

[People] ought to know that from the brain, and from the brain only, arise our pleasures, joys, laughter and jests, as well as our sorrows, pains, griefs and tears. Through it, in particular, we think, see, hear, and distinguish the ugly from the beautiful, the bad from the good, the pleasant from the unpleasant.... It is the same thing which makes us mad or delirious, inspires us with dread and fear, whether by night or by day, brings sleeplessness, inopportune mistakes, aimless anxieties, absent-mindedness, and acts that are contrary to habit. These things that we suffer all come from the brain, when it is not healthy, but becomes abnormally hot, cold, moist, or dry, or suffers any other unnatural affection to which it was not accustomed. Madness comes from its moisture. When the brain is abnormally moist, of necessity it moves, and when it moves, neither sight nor hearing are still, but we see or hear now one thing and now another, and the tongue speaks in accordance with the things seen and heard on any occasion. But all the time the brain is still, a man can think properly.

Attributed to HIPPOCRATES,
Fifth century BC
From Eric Kandel and James Schwartz,
Principles of Neural Science, 2nd ed., 1985

SENTIENCE

Sentient: 1. having sense perception; conscious 2. experiencing
sensation or feeling [Latin: present participle of *sentire*, to feel.
Root *sent*—to head for, to go (i.e., to go mentally)]

AMERICAN HERITAGE DICTIONARY OF THE
ENGLISH LANGUAGE

Have you ever noticed that everything about you is perfect, in the
sense of being perfectly as and what it already is? Consider for a
moment: like everybody else, you are born, you develop, you grow
up, you live your life, make your choices, have the things that happen to you happen to you for better or for worse. Ultimately, if your
life is not abruptly foreshortened, or even if it is, you have dealt with
what you could. You have done your work, contributed in one way or
another, left your legacy. You have been in relationships with others
and with the world, and perhaps tasted or bathed in love and shared
yours with the world. Inexorably, you age and, if you are lucky, grow
older—with the emphasis on the growing—continuing to share your
being with others and with the world in any number of ways, satisfying or not. And finally, you die.

It has happened to everybody who has ever lived on this planet. It
will happen to me. It will happen to you. This is the human condition.

But it is not all of it.

The bird's-eye, boiled-down view I have just sketched out is woefully incomplete, although it is not meant to be a caricature. For there is another invisible element that is co-extensive with our life and critical to its unfolding yet so woven into the fabric of all our moments, so obvious, that we hardly ever consider it. All the same, it is that essence that makes us not only what we are, but bestows upon us a largeness of capacity we so infrequently even sense, never mind honor and develop to its full expression. I am speaking, of course, about awareness, about what is called sentience, our ability to know; our consciousness; our subjective experience.

For we have, after all, named our very species and genus *Homo sapiens sapiens* (a double dose of the present participle of *sapere*, to taste; to perceive; to know; to be wise). The implication is quite clear. What we think differentiates us from other species is our ability to be wise in our perceiving, to be knowing, and to be aware of our knowing. But this characteristic is also so taken for granted by us in our ordinary everyday lives that it remains virtually unseen, unknown, or at best, only vaguely appreciated. We don't make maximum advantage of our sentience when, in fact, it defines us in virtually every moment of our waking and dreaming lives.

It is sentience that animates us. It is the ultimate mystery, that which makes us more than a mere mechanism that thinks and feels. We are perceivers, yes, like all beings, yet we are capable of a discerning and discriminating wisdom beyond mere perception, a gift that may be uniquely ours on this small world. Our sentience defines our possibilities but in no way delimits the boundaries of the possible for us. We are the species that grows into itself. We are creatures who are forever learning and, as a consequence, modulating both ourselves and the world. And as a developing species, we have come to all this in a remarkably short period of time.

At the moment, neuroscientists know a lot about the brain and the mind, and more every day. Still, they have no understanding whatsoever of sentience and how it comes about. It is a huge conundrum, a mystery that seems unfathomable. Matter arranged in a complex enough way can evidently hold the world "in mind" as we say, and know it. Mind appears. Consciousness arises. And we have no idea how. In cognitive neuroscience, this is known as "the hard problem."

It is one thing to have upside-down two-dimensional images on the backs of our retinas. It is quite another to see: to have a vivid experience of a world existing "out there" in three dimensions, beyond our own body, a world that seems real, and that we can sense, move in, and be conscious of, and even conjure up in the mind in great detail with our eyes closed. And within this conjuring, somehow, a sense of personhood is generated as well, a sense of a seer who is doing the seeing and perceiving what is to be seen, a knower who is knowing what is here to be known, at least to a degree. Yet it is all a conjuring, a construct of the mind, literally a fabrication, a synthesizing of a world out of sensory input, a synthesis based at least in part on processing vast arrays of sensory information through complex networks in the brain, the whole of the nervous system, and indeed, the whole of the body. This is truly a phenomenal accomplishment. It is a huge mystery, and an extraordinary, if usually entirely taken for granted, inheritance for each of us.

Sir Francis Crick, neurobiologist and co-discoverer of the double helical structure of DNA, observed that "…in spite of all this work [in the psychology, physiology, molecular and cell biology of vision], we really have no clear idea how we see anything." Even the color blue (or any other color) does not exist either in the photons that make up the light of that particular wavelength nor anywhere in the eye or brain. Yet we look up at a cloudless sky on a sunny day and know that it is blue. And if we have no clear idea how we see anything, that is even more the case for understanding, physiologically speaking, how we know anything.

Steven Pinker, linguist and evolutionary neuropsychologist, in his book, *How the Mind Works*, writes about sentience as a phenomenon apart, in a class by itself:

In the study of mind, sentience floats in its own plane, high above the causal chains of physiology and neuroscience.... we cannot banish sentience from our discourse or reduce it to information access, because moral reasoning depends on it. The concept of sentience underlies our certainty that torture is wrong, and that disabling a robot is the destruction of property but disabling a person is murder. It is the reason that the death of a loved one does not impart to us just self-pity at our loss but the uncomprehending pain of knowing that the person's thoughts and pleasures have vanished forever.

Yet Crick asserts that, whatever it is, sentience, and the sense of agency we link to the pronouns "I" and "me," like every other quality, phenomenon, and experience we associate with mind, is ultimately due to the activity of neurons, an emergent phenomenon of brain structure and activity behind which there is no agent, only neuro-electrical and neuro-chemical impulses:

The mental picture most of us have is that there is a little man (or woman) somewhere inside our brain who is following (or, at least, trying hard to follow) what is going on. I shall call this the Fallacy of the Homunculus (*homunculus* is Latin for "little man"). Many people do indeed feel this way—and that fact, in due course will itself need an explanation—but our Astonishing Hypothesis states that this is not the case. Loosely speaking, it says that "it's all done by neurons...." There must be structures or operations in the brain that, in some mysterious way, behave as if they correspond somewhat to the mental picture of the homunculus.

To which the philosopher John Searle responds: "How is it possible for physical, objective, quantitatively describable neuron firings to cause qualitative, private, subjective experiences?" This is a big challenge in the field of robotics, where researchers are attempting to make machines that do things, such as mowing the lawn when it needs mowing, or putting away the dishes when they are clean, things that we can do without a moment's thought (we say) but are incredibly difficult problems for robots to solve. And beyond that, as we have seen, in the exploding field of AI (artificial intelligence), machines designed by us are now designing and constructing (or at least contributing to the construction of) the next generations of machines. With each iteration, the newly designed machines increase their complexity and "learn" as they go along. At some point it begins to look and feel as if the machines themselves have feelings and are actually thinking, accomplishing this with integrated circuits rather than with neurons but all the same, at least seeming to mimic or simulate what we would say looks and feels a lot like agency, intelligence, and emotion. And of course, in some sense it may be that we ourselves could actually be elaborate "receivers," tuning in because of our neurons, to a much higher-order non-local "mind" that is a property of the universe. Some people think that possibility cannot be entirely ruled out at present.

Our challenge here is not to wander too far afield into various explanations for sentience and the scientific and philosophical controversies presently surrounding it, fascinating as this inquiry and the scientific and philosophical domains that concern themselves with such questions, such as cognitive neuroscience, phenomenology, artificial intelligence, and so-called neuro-phenomenology, are. Rather, our challenge is more basic and closer to home, namely to recognize our sentience as fundamental and to ponder whether it might serve us individually and collectively to *develop* this extraordinary capacity for knowing which, remarkably and importantly, includes of course innumerable occasions for knowing that we don't know. Knowing that we don't know is just as important, if not more so, than anything else we might know. Here lies the domain of discernment and wisdom, in a sense we might say, the quintessence of being human.

At the end of a retreat for psychologists training in mindfulness-based cognitive therapy, one therapist, who of course works with people and their emotions and thoughts all day long, said: "I wall myself off from people. It was something I didn't know I didn't know."

Our lives are all too often lived out under the constraints of habits and conditioning that we are entirely unaware of but which shape our moments and our choices, our experiences, and our emotional responses to them, even when we think we know better, or should know better. This alone suggests some of the practical limitations of thinking.

Yet amazingly, awareness itself, the whole domain of sentience and multiple intelligences, is continually available to us to counter that conditioning and expand our feeling for things, allowing us to be more in touch with them and with our capacity for actually understanding what the neuroscientist Antonio Damasio calls "the feeling of what happens."

Sentience is closer than close. Awareness is our nature and is in our nature. It is in our bodies, in our species. It could be said, as the Tibetans do, that cognizance, the non-conceptual *knowing* quality, is the essence of what we call mind, along with emptiness and boundlessness, which Tibetan Buddhism sees as complementary aspects of the very same essence.

The capacity for awareness appears to be built into us. We can't help but be aware. It is the defining characteristic of our species. Grounded in our biology, it extends far beyond the merely biological. It is what and who we actually are. Yet, if not cultivated and refined, and in some ways even protected, our capacity for sentience tends to get covered over by tangles of vines and underbrush and remain weak and undeveloped, in some ways merely a potential. We can become relatively insensate, insensitive, more asleep than awake when it comes to drawing on our ability to know beyond the limitations of self-serving thought—and which would include the recognizing of thoughts that are self-serving and therefore knowing that they may be limited and potentially unwise in the very moments in which they arise. Cultivated and strengthened, sentience lights up our lives and it lights up the world, and grants us degrees of freedom we could scarcely imagine even though our imagination itself stems from it.

It also grants us a wisdom that, developed, can steer us clear of our tendencies to cause harm, wittingly or unwittingly, and instead, can soothe the wounds and honor the sovereignty and the sanctity of fellow sentient beings everywhere.

Nothing Personal, But, Excuse Me . . . Are We Who We Think We Are?

The true value of a human being is determined primarily by the measure and the sense in which he has attained liberation from the self.

Albert Einstein

As biology students, it was hammered into us (this is one of a number of metaphors that are not uncommon within higher education) that life obeys the laws of physics and chemistry and that biological phenomena are merely an extension of those same natural laws; that while life is complex, and the molecules of life far more elaborate than the simpler atomic and molecular structures of inanimate nature and in more dynamic relationship to one another, there is no reason to suspect that there is some extra special animating or "vital" force that is "causing" the whole system to be alive; nothing special, that is, beyond the mix of fairly sensitive conditions that permit the components and structures of living systems to act in concert somehow to allow the properties of the whole to emerge as, say, a living, growing, dividing cell. By extension, the same principle would apply throughout the web of increasingly complex life forms branching out into the plant and animal kingdoms including, in our mammalian lineage, the emergence of increasingly complex nervous systems, and, in time, the advent of ourselves.

Said another way, this view affirms that while we do not fully understand what we call "life" even at the level of one single cell, even at the level of a very "simple," single-cell organism such as a bacterium, there is no inherent reason that this could not be done, and indeed, an entirely synthetic bacterium was created in 2010. Earlier, in a similar breakthrough, researchers synthesized the polio virus from scratch out of simple chemicals and information about the virus's genetic sequence obtained off the Internet. Once made, it was shown to be infectious and able to replicate and make more virus in a living cell, thereby demonstrating that no "extra" vital force was necessary. Of course, ethical issues associated with such work are huge.

This perspective, that there is no "extra" nonmaterial animating element to living systems, stands in biology as a revered bulwark against what used to be called vitalism, the belief that some special energy other than natural processes explainable through physics, chemistry, biology, natural selection, and a huge amount of time, is required to give life its unique properties. And that would include sentience. Vitalism was seen as mystical, irrational, anti-scientific, and just plain wrong. And in the historical record, of course, it was and is just plain wrong. But that doesn't mean that a reductionist and purely materialist perspective is necessarily right. There are multiple ways of exploring and understanding the mystery of life through scientific inquiry, ways that take into account and respect higher orders of phenomena, and their emergent properties.

From the biological perspective, there is nothing but impersonal mechanism at the very base of living systems, including us. It sees the emergence of life itself as an extension of a larger emergence, the evolution of the entire universe and all the ordered structures and processes that unfold within it. At some point, perhaps around three billion years ago, when the conditions were right on the young planet Earth—which had formed out of the interstellar dust cloud surrounding the nascent star we call our sun, that dust itself being the result of the colossal disintegration via gravitational collapse of earlier stars in which the very atoms, the atomic elements, except for hydrogen, that constitute our bodies and everything else on this planet were forged—biomolecules couldn't help but be synthesized by naturally occurring inorganic processes in warm pools and oceans over millions and millions of years, perhaps catalyzed by lightning, by clays, and other inanimate microenvironments that could contribute in various ways to such processes. Given enough time, these various ingredients found ways to interact according to the laws of chemistry to give rise to rudimentary polymer chains of nucleotides (the stuff of DNA and RNA) and amino acids that had particular properties.

By their very nature, polynucleotide chains have the capacity to store huge amounts of information in the sequence of their four constituent bases, to self-replicate with high precision to conserve that information, and to change slightly under various conditions and thus produce variants, known as mutations that may, rarely, have a selective advantage in competing for natural resources. This information in the polynucleotide chains is translated into the linear sequence of amino acids that constitute poly-amino acid chains that, when they fold up, are known as proteins, the workhorses of the cell that perform all its thousands of chemical reactions, in which case they are called enzymes, and that provide a myriad of key structural building blocks out of which cells are made, in which case they are known as structural proteins.

How it all came about to give rise to an organized cell in the first place, even an exceedingly primitive one, is not understood. But from the perspective of biology, in principle it can and will be understood, and all that will be necessary to understand it will be deeper insight into complex systems of such molecules that themselves have no vital force other than the capacity, under the right conditions and in concert with many other such molecules, for the unpredictable emergence

of novel phenomena, including, importantly, the stabilizing, st
ing, and retrieval of information and the modulation of its flow. In
this sense, life is a natural extension of the evolution of the universe,
once stars and planets are created that allow the conditions necessary for chemistry-based living systems to emerge. And consciousness, which emerges within living systems following those same laws
of physics and chemistry when the conditions are friendly to it and
there is enough time and selective pressure for that level of complexity
to develop, is also therefore seen as a natural, if highly improbable,
emergence from a biological evolutionary process that is empty of a
driving force, empty of teleology, not at all mystical.

If consciousness, at least chemistry-based consciousness, is built
in as potentially possible or even inevitable in an evolving universe
given the correct initial conditions and enough time, one might say,
as we have noted already, that consciousness in living organisms is a
way for the universe to know itself, to see itself, even to understand
itself. We could say that in this local neighborhood of the vastness
of it all, that gift has fallen to us, to *Homo sapiens sapiens*, apparently
more so than to any other species on this infinitesimally small speck
we inhabit in the unimaginable vastness of the expanding universe,
where our kind of matter, that makes up our bodies and the planets
and even all the stars, seems to account for only a tiny percentage of
the substance and energy of the universe.* In this view, our capacity
for consciousness has fallen to us not because of any particular moral
virtue but purely by accident, by the vagaries of evolutionary selection
pressures on tree-dwelling primate species, some of which evolved to
stand erect as they moved onto the savannah and freed up the use of

---

* Indeed, cosmologists now view the universe as consisting of about 30 percent "dark
matter," perhaps sequestered in black holes, and of greater than 65 percent "dark energy,"
which may be responsible for the pervading force behind the universe's accelerating
expansion, a kind of anti-gravity.

their arms and hands and gave their brains a greater range of challenges to deal with. These, of course, were our direct ancestors.

How we understand our inherited sentience and what we do with it individually and collectively as a species is clearly the defining issue of our time. The impersonal nature of the biological view of living systems is worth emphasizing, because it says very clearly that there is no intrinsically mystical dimension to the unfolding of life. It says that consciousness does not direct the process but emerges out of the process, even though the potential for its emergence was latent all the time. Nevertheless, once consciousness emerges and is refined, it can have a profound influence on all aspects of life, through the choices that we make about how to live and where to place our energies, and how to appreciate our impact in and on the world we inhabit. Sentience could only emerge given the right causes and conditions, which are not guaranteed to happen. Of course, if they hadn't, there wouldn't have been any of us around to comment on its absence in any event.

If we ourselves are the product of impersonal causes and conditions following on the laws of physics and chemistry, however complex, and if there is no "vital force" behind it all, then we can see why the anti-vitalism of science, especially biology, would lead to the declaring that there is no such thing as a soul, a vital center within a sentient being that is following laws other than the laws of physics and chemistry. In the seventeenth century, Descartes declared the seat of the soul to be in the pineal gland deep in the brain. Modern neurobiologists would say that the pineal gland may do many things but it does not generate a soul because there is no reason to postulate an enduring entity or energy that is immaterial and that inhabits or interfaces with the organism in some way and guides its trajectory through life. That doesn't mean that life and sentience are not hugely mysterious to us, or for that matter, sacred, just as the universe itself is hugely mysterious. Nor does it mean that we can't speak of the soul, meaning what moves deeply in the psyche and in the heart, nor of the source of uplift and transfiguration we call spirit. It also does not imply that one's personal feelings and personal well-being are not important, or that there is no basis for ethical or moral action, or for that matter, a sense of the numinous. In fact, we could say that it is our nature and calling as sentient beings to regard our situation with awe and wonder, and to wonder deeply about the potential for exploring and refining our sentience and placing it in the service of the well-being of others, and of what is most beautiful and indeed most sacred in this living world—so sacred that we would guard ourselves much more effectively than we have so far from causing it—the world that is—to be disregarded or perhaps even destroyed by our own precocity.

Buddhists hold a similar view of the fundamentally impersonal nature of phenomena. As we encountered in the Heart Sutra (see Book 1, *Meditation Is Not What You Think*, "Emptiness"), the Buddha taught, based on his own personal investigations and experience, that the entire world that can be experienced—what he termed the five *skandas* (heaps): forms, feelings, perceptions, impulses, and consciousness—is empty of any enduring self-existing characteristic; that try as one might, one will not be able to locate a permanent, unchanging self-ness inside or underneath any phenomenon, living or inanimate, including ourselves, because everything is interconnected and each manifestation of form or process depends on a constantly changing web of causes and conditions for its individual emergence and its particular properties. He challenges us to look and see for ourselves and investigate whether or not it is so, whether or not the self is merely a fabrication, a construct, just as in some way our senses combine to construct both the world that appears to be "out there" and the sense of the person "in here" that perceives it.

Well, if it is not so, then how is it that we *feel* that there is a self, that we are a self, that what happens happens to a me, that what I do is initiated by me, what I feel is felt by me, that when I wake up in the morning, it is the same me waking up and recognizing myself in the mirror? Both modern biology (cognitive neuroscience) and

Buddhism would say that it is something of a mis-perception that has built itself into an enduring individual and cultural habit. Nevertheless, if you go through the process of systematically searching for it, they hold that you will not find a permanent, independent, enduring self, whether you look for it in "your" body, including its cells, specialized glands, nervous system, brain, and so forth, in "your" emotions, "your" beliefs, "your" thoughts, "your" relationships, or anyplace else. And the reason you will not be able to locate anywhere a permanent, isolated, self-existing self that is "you" is that it is a mirage, a holographic emergence, a phantom, a product of the habit-bound, emotionally turbulent, thinking mind. It is being constructed and deconstructed continually, moment by moment. It is continually subject to change, and therefore not permanent or enduring or real, in the sense of identifiable and isolatable. It is more virtual than solid, akin at least metaphorically to virtual elementary particles that appear to emerge out of nothing for a brief moment in the quantum foam of empty space and then dissolve back into the nothing. Or what we call the self could also be described as a "strange attractor" in the world of chaos theory, a dynamical pattern that is continually changing but is always self-similar. You are who you were yesterday, more or less, but not exactly.

To play with this a little bit more, let's look at what we mean when we refer to "my" body. Who is saying this? Who exactly is claiming to have a body, and is therefore separate from that very body? It is rather mysterious, isn't it? Our language itself is self-referential. It requires that we say "my body" (just count the number of times on this page, or even in this sentence, that I have had to use personal pronouns to say anything about us), and we get in the habit of thinking that that is who we are, or at least a large part of who we are. It becomes an unquestioned part of our conventional reality. Of course, at the level of appearances, it *is* the case, relatively speaking.

Most of the time, we wouldn't say "the" hand, or "the" leg or "the" head, we would say "my," because, relatively speaking, this body of ours (there I go again) is in some relationship to the speaker, whoever that is, and referring to it as "the" hand would seem distanced, alienated, somehow clinical and disembodied. Nonetheless, there is a mysterious relationship between me and my body, but one that usually goes totally unexamined. Because it is unexamined, it is easy to fall into believing that it is "my" body without even knowing that we don't exactly know who is claiming that ownership, and that it is only a convenient way of speaking rather than a fact. It is relatively so (after all, it is not somebody else's body—that kind of thinking or feeling can be severely pathological and would put you on a course for hospitalization) but it is not so in an absolute way. If what the Heart Sutra says is accurate, appearance itself is empty.

The same is true for the mind. Whose mind is it? And who has trouble making it up? And who wants to know? Who is reading these words?

Imagine for a moment that what the biologists and the Buddhists say is true (although for the Buddhists, mind is another dimensionality that follows its own lawfulness, which can be related to material phenomena, i.e., a brain, but is not reducible to matter). As a living being, we would be the product of chemistry and physics and biology, and of wholly impersonal processes that give rise to our experience as we interface with the world beyond our skin, and with the milieu of the body and mind. The sense of a self, of a "me" to whom all these experiences are happening, and who is thinking these thoughts, feeling these feelings, making these decisions, and acting this way or that is, if anything, an epi-phenomenon, a by-product of complex biological processes. Both the sense of personhood and our personality are in a profound way impersonal, although clearly unique and relatively real, even as one's face is unique and relatively real but not anywhere near the whole story of who we are.

If that were so, what would we lose, and what might be gained from a radical shift in perspective on ourselves to a larger, more expansive and perhaps more fundamental view?

What would be lost would be an overly strong identification with virtually all experience, inward and outward, as "I," "me," and "mine," instead of as impersonal phenomena that unfold according to various causes and conditions or, you could say, that just happen. If we can learn to question the ways in which a sense of a self solidifies around occurrences and appearances and then defends itself at all costs, if we choose to question whether the sense of self is fundamentally real or just a construct of mind, to examine whether it is invariant or continually changing, and to ponder even how important its views are in any moment in relationship to the larger whole, then we might not be so self-preoccupied and consumed so much of the time with our thoughts and opinions and with our personal stories of gain and loss, and so strongly oriented toward maximizing the former and minimizing the latter. We might see through this veil of our own creation that subtly or not so subtly colors every aspect of experience. We might hear ourselves more accurately. We might take ourselves less seriously, and we might take less seriously the stories we concoct about how things should be for me to be happy or to get "my way." We might take less personally things that are fundamentally not personal.

Were we to do so, there might also be more of a sense of ease in inhabiting the body and in living in the world, more of a sense of wonder at the very fact of being and being alive, the very fact of knowing, without having to get caught up so much in that fixed sense of a "knower" that splits off from what is known, creating both subject (a me) and objects out there (to be known by me), and a distance between them rather than an intimacy in their reciprocity, a co-arising with awareness, in awareness. Imagine if we were a little less self-absorbed in those ways, not having to push our own small agenda because we see and know that that very sense of self is empty of inherent existence; that it has only an appearance of existing, and that a strong identification with it locks us into a warped, diminished, and seriously incomplete view of our being, of our life, especially in relationship to the lives of others, and of our path in this world.

For one thing, perhaps you have noticed that the sense of self is telling us all the time that we are not complete. It tells us that we have to get someplace else, attain what needs to be achieved, become whole, become happy, make a difference, get on with it, all of which may indeed be partially true and relatively true, and to that degree, we need to honor those intuitions. But it forgets to remind us that, on a deeper level, beyond appearances and time, whatever needs to be attained is already here, now—that there is no improving the self—only knowing its true nature as both empty and full, and therefore complete, whole as it is, and also profoundly useful.

Knowing this in the deepest of ways, knowing it with the entirety of our being, a capacity which develops with ongoing mindfulness practice, we can then rest in the knowing itself and act much less self-centeredly in the world for the benefit of other beings, and with an attitude of non-harming and non-forcing. We can do this because we know on some fundamental level, not merely intellectually, that "them" is always "us." This interconnectedness is primary. It is the birthplace of empathy and compassion, of our feeling for the other, our impulse and tendency to put ourself in the place of the other, to feel with the other. This is the foundation for ethics and morality, for becoming fully human—beyond the potential nihilism and groundless relativism stemming from a merely mechanistic and reductionist view of the mind and of life.

From this perspective, in a very real sense you are not who or what you think you are. And neither is anybody else. We are all much larger and more mysterious. Once we know this, our possibilities for creativity expand enormously because we understand something about how habitually we wind up getting in our own way, and are diminished through our obsessive self-involvement and self-centeredness, our preoccupation with what we think is important but isn't really fundamental.

It's not a criticism. It's just a fact.
Nothing personal, so please don't take it that way.

*

I am not I.
   I am this one
Walking beside me whom I do not see,
Whom at times I manage to visit,
And whom at other times I forget...

JUAN RAMON JIMÉNEZ
Translated by Robert Bly

*

Enough. These few words are enough.
If not these words, this breath.
If not this breath, this sitting here.

This opening to the life
we have refused
again and again
until now.

Until now.

DAVID WHYTE

EVEN OUR MOLECULES TOUCH

Francisco Varela, polymath cognitive neuroscientist, neuro-phenomenologist philosopher, and dedicated dharma practitioner, co-founder of the Mind and Life Institute, which holds periodic dialogues between scientists and the Dalai Lama, died at the age of 54 in 2001. Francisco used to emphasize those properties of the immune system that transcended its role as an effective defense system against outside invaders. For the immune system also serves as a self-sensing system, with mechanisms that allow the body continually to monitor and affirm its "self-ness," the utterly unique molecular identity of all its constituent structures, through molecular touching. At the same time, Francisco emphasized that this self-quality that we could call "my" bodily identity doesn't actually have an independent existence any more than we do, but emerges dynamically out of the complex interactions among its constituent parts.

Sometimes the immune system is referred to as the body's second brain because it is capable of learning and changing and remembering in response to changing conditions. Anatomically, it is partially localized in the thymus, the bone marrow, and the spleen, and in part, it is non-localized, in that its lymphocytes and the antibody molecules they produce can circulate independently in the blood and lymph. Lymphocytes have specialized receptor molecules (including antibodies) embedded in their membranes which allow them to "feel" the contours and architecture of the body at the molecular level, the topology of its circulating molecules, its cells, its organs, and its tissues, and thus know itself and identify non-self "foreign invaders" through continual surveillance and mechanisms for highly specific molecular recognition.

Even in the absence of foreign invaders or disease processes, there seems to be a continual conversation among all the members of the society of cells that constitutes the body, carried on through the language of immune signaling and recognition. The conversation coordinates all the various functions of the body on a cellular level. Without it, even in the absence of infection, the body would degrade. As Varela put it:

> The sense organs that relate the brain to the environment, such as the eyes and ears, have parallels in a number of lymph organs. These are distinct regions that act as sensing devices and interact with stimuli: for example, patches in the intestine that constantly relate to what you eat.

When something does go awry, if certain cells mutate and start growing out of control, or strange viral particles or other substances appear in the body, these are detected, sensed, "felt" by the touch recognition systems of the immune system. Then, various cell-based and antibody-based mechanisms are mobilized to contain and neutralize them with an amazing degree of specificity based on clonal selection and amplification of those lymphocytes that deploy the specific recognition molecules in question so that the abnormal cells or chemicals are neutralized while normal cells are not attacked or harmed.

The immune system is a beehive of selective touching and recognition, a surveillance system that never sleeps so that harmony is maintained in the dynamic life field of the body as it is exposed to potentially damaging agents from within and without. It functions with an exquisite elegance on both the molecular and cellular levels to allow the body to respond to threats it has never before seen, whether from infectious agents or from man-made compounds that didn't exist on the planet when human beings were evolving and yet can be recognized as potentially damaging, sequestered and neutralized. This response is learned and then remembered by the immune system.

When this system breaks down, as it sometimes mysteriously does, you lose the protective recognition of the bodily self. That gives rise to the so-called autoimmune diseases, where the immune system now attacks the normal tissues of the body. The members of the society of cells and tissues that make up the body are no longer in touch with one another in ways that optimize harmony and health. The conversations among them either dissolve or turn toxic. This is not that different than when social groupings and nations cease being able to find common ground.

Regarding the question of bodily identity and the role of the immune system beyond that of defense, Francisco used a social analogy to give a feeling for its non-self-existing nature. Since he lived in Paris, he used France as an example. Here is Francisco, speaking to the Dalai Lama:

What is the nature of the identity of a nation? France, for example, has an identity, and it is not sitting in the office of François Mitterrand [this conversation took place in 1990, when Mitterrand was president of France]. Obviously, if too much of a foreign entity invades the system, it will have outer-directed defense reactions. The army mounts a military response; however, it would be silly to say that the military response is the whole of French identity. What is the identity of France when there is no war? Communication creates this identity, the tissue of social life, as people meet each other and talk. It is the life beat of the country. You walk in the cities and see people in cafés, writing books, raising children, cooking—but most of all, talking. Something analogous happens in the immune system as we construct our bodily identity. Cells and tissues have an identity

as a body because of the network of B-cells and T-cells constantly moving around, binding and unbinding, to every single molecular profile in your body. They also bind and unbind
constantly *among themselves*. A large percent of a B-cell's con-
tacts are with other B-cells. Like a society, the cells build a
tissue of mutual interactions, a functional network...And
it is through these mutual interactions that lymphocytes are
inhibited or expanded in clones, just as people get demoted
or promoted, families expand or contract. This affirmation
of a system's identity, which is not a defensive reaction but a
positive construction, is a kind of self-assertion. This is what
constitutes our "self" on the molecular and cellular level...
There are T-cells that can bind to every single molecular
profile in the body, just as for every aspect of French life—
museums and libraries, cafés and pastries—there must be
people who deal with it...The fact is, you do find antibodies
to every single molecular profile in your body (cell membrane,
muscle proteins, hormones, and so on)...Through this dis-
tributed interdependence, a global balance is created, so that
the molecules of my skin are in communication with the cells
in my liver, because they are mutually affected via this circulating network of the immune system. From the perspective
of network immunology, the immune system is nothing other
than an enabler of the constant communication between
every cell in your body, much as neurons link distant places
in the nervous system...The cells of the immune system die
and are replaced roughly every two days [although some live
much longer, weeks and even months], just as in a society,
people die after a number of years and children are constantly
being born. Society in some complex way trains this pool of
children to fill different roles. This is how the system renews
its components. Learning, or memory, happens because new
cells are being "educated" into the system. The new cells are

not identical to the old ones, but they fill the same role for the overall purpose of the emergent global picture...

We are not used to thinking of the body as a self that is as complex an entity as our cognitive selves, but the fact is that we do function that way... Going back to the social analogy, I buy my bread every day from a baker in Paris whose family has been there for 200 years. He's part of the society, and he knows how to bake his bread. If suddenly one day I find a different person at the same bakery, who may be doing the same actions, selling the same bread, it still won't be the same. The baker belongs there because of the history of his long interactions, the fact that he's known people for a long time, and they have a common language. You can imitate this French baker, but if you don't have the right history and language and the capacity to interact, the neighbors will reject you too. What establishes my cells in their places and allows my liver cells to behave as liver cells, my thymus cells to behave as thymus cells, and so on, is the fact that they share this common language so they can operate in context with each other. Similarly, the baker knows the banker belongs to the community, even though the banker is doing something different. We are so used to our body working that we don't appreciate the complexity of this emerging process that maintains its working. Much as in the human brain, where capacities such as memory or a sense of self are emergent properties of all the neurons, in the immune system there is an emergent capacity to maintain the body, and to have a history with it, to have a self. As an emergent property, it is something that arises but doesn't exist anywhere... My bodily identity is not localized in my genes or in my cells, but in the complex of interactions.

This vital, dynamic perspective will be worth keeping in mind when we explore the metaphor of the world as one body in Book 4.

No Fragmentation

As you may have experienced by now to some degree, just in paying a bit more careful attention to the activity of your own mind and body from moment to moment, and perhaps even more so if you have by now taken up the formal practice of mindfulness meditation, that we tend to lead rather fragmented lives, both inwardly and outwardly. And we contribute to and participate in this fragmentation through a temporary forgetting of who we actually are in our deepest nature, and by our impulse to be not as we are but as others, or even our own fantasizing, would have us be. Thus, we split ourselves off from ourselves. We fragment ourselves to pursue chimera, often for years and decades at a stretch, and in the process, lose touch with or even betray at times our true nature, our sovereignty, the beauty of who we actually are, and our unfragmented, unfragmentable wholeness. This is one symptom of our endemic distress and dis-ease both as individuals and as a society. Perhaps this splitting ourselves off from ourselves is the root conflict. Perhaps it lies at the core of all conflict.

Healing is a process; one that involves the recognition of our wholeness, and a steadfast refusal to allow ourselves to be fragmented, even when we are terrified or broken apart by life. Ultimately, healing is a coming to terms with things as they are, rather than struggling to force them to be as they once were, or as we would like them to be to feel secure, or to have what we sometimes think of as our own way. As my colleague and friend Saki Santorelli puts it, healing is a matter of knowing that we can be shattered and yet still whole.

Emily Dickinson was able to capture so utterly poignantly this endemic impulse to split off parts of ourselves, to fragment in the face of our own fear, and wounds:

Me from Myself—to banish—
Had I Art—
Impregnable my Fortress
Unto All Heart—

But since Myself—assault Me—
How have I peace
Except by subjugating
Consciousness?

And since We're mutual Monarch
How this be
Except by Abdication—
Me—of Me?

How often do we voluntarily but unwittingly banish ourselves from ourselves, abdicate our wholeness, and subjugate our consciousness, our sentience, and our common sense, our very sovereignty and the possibilities of true healing, in the hope of achieving invulnerability, to protect ourselves from more hurt, to lessen our pain?

What is the price we pay for such abdication? Is it worth it?

What if we were to choose, bravely, not to subjugate our consciousness any longer? Or even for just one moment?

Who would we be?

How might we feel, inwardly?

How might we act, outwardly?

No Separation

Einstein, who in his time saw far more deeply than others into the nature of space and time, matter and energy, light and gravitation, also saw, perhaps equally deeply, into the blinding effects of desire and attachment and how important it is to dissolve what he called the delusion of separateness. Responding to a rabbi who had written explaining that he had thought in vain to comfort his nineteen-year-old daughter over the death of her sister, a "sinless, beautiful sixteen-year-old child,"* Einstein replied:

A human being is a part of the whole, called by us "Universe," a part limited in time and space. He experiences himself, his thoughts and feelings as something separated from the rest— a kind of optical delusion of his consciousness. This delusion is a kind of prison for us, restricting us to our personal desires and to affection for a few persons nearest to us. Our task must be to free ourselves from this prison by widening our circle of compassion to embrace all living creatures and the whole nature in its beauty. Nobody is able to achieve this completely, but the striving for such achievement is in itself a part of the liberation, and a foundation for inner security.

That Einstein, a great physicist, also thought in terms of liberation

* *New York Times*: March 29, 1972.

and inner security is in itself hugely telling. It underscores how much he felt we are all plagued by the delusion of separation, the separation of me from myself, and me from you, and I from Thou, how much he understood the suffering that stems from it, and the need to guard against it by cultivating compassion.

He saw in terms of wholes, with eyes of wholeness. And in terms of liberation from delusion. And his response was... compassion.

Can we ask ourselves to see with eyes of wholeness as well, and be aware of the prisons we create for ourselves and for others through our delusions of separation when fundamentally there really is none? Can we, as Einstein put it, widen our circle of compassion to "embrace all living creatures and the whole nature in its beauty"? And can we include ourselves in that circle of compassion?

Why not?

It is a practice, after all, not a philosophy. And that practice is called waking up from the delusions, the fragmentations, the abdications, the fabrications of our own mis-perceptions; it is called freeing ourselves from what appears to be "apartness" when in fact, at the deepest of levels, we truly belong, have always been seamlessly woven into the whole, are already at home, here, in this moment, with this breath, in this place.

*

Ah, not to be cut off,
not through the slightest partition
shut out from the law of the stars.
The inner—what is it?
if not intensified sky,
hurled through with birds and deep
with the winds of homecoming.

RILKE
Translated by Stephen Mitchell

Orienting in Time and Space:
A Tribute to My Father

Who am I? Where am I? What time is it? Where was I? What was I doing? Where am I going?

No, this is not the title of a Gauguin painting, although it might be.

But these are fundamental questions. We count ourselves lucky if we can remember to shut off the stove after using it, and then some time later recall that we actually did shut it off, which is harder. But we hardly ever feel lucky to know what we are doing, or who we are, or where we are, or what time it is. We should. We take an awful lot for granted that is quite miraculous, enlivening, and that gives meaning to every unfolding moment of our lives.

As my father was gradually losing large swatches of his mind to Alzheimer's disease, I became disturbingly aware of how much I took for granted. I knew where I was, how I got there, what had come before, what might be coming next. It was not that I had to think about it at all. I just knew. All of that was dissolving for him. It was as if huge holes were opening up in his brain. Time and place and causality were among the early casualties.

My father, Elvin Kabat, had spent his entire career at Columbia University Medical Center, except for a twenty-year stretch toward the end of it when he had, amazingly for a man of his age, commuted back and forth each week between his lab in New York and a project he oversaw at the National Institutes of Health in Bethesda,

Maryland, which involved compiling, putting online, and continually updating the sequences of all known antibody molecules and later of their genes.

One day, a colleague of his from Columbia called me to recount the following: Toward the end of having lunch together in the doctors' dining room, my father mentioned that he was heading off to the airport to go back to New York. The problem was, he was already in New York. By the time of that phone call, my family and I already knew.

The first episode that I allowed to, or more accurately, which I couldn't prevent penetrating my consciousness occurred when he declared with some glee that, in doing his taxes that year, which he had always done himself, he was getting the IRS to reimburse him for all his travel between New York and the NIH. (I would have thought it was already paid for out of his grants.) But inconceivably, he was confusing a deduction with a reimbursement. I was shattered. I remember to this day the sinking feeling that arose somewhere deep in my chest and descended sickeningly into my stomach as the reality of that realization took effect. This was of a different order entirely from not being able to come up with a word, or forgetting where he put his keys.

Could this be happening? What did this portend for my father, whose own mentor, the great immunologist Michael Heidelberger, had lived to be 103 and who had shown up in his lab every day to meet with students and to write scientific papers until he was 102. My father's one desire, which he clung to more and more as he felt himself aging, was that he remain creative and continue to do what he called "productive work" in his beloved laboratory. For his entire life he had lived almost exclusively in and by his mind, blessed with an iron will and razor-sharp intellect. He held an endowed chair in microbiology, was a professor in three other departments, and was a Presidential Medal of Science winner for his pioneering work in immunochemistry and molecular immunology. He was a long-standing member of the National Academy of Sciences, a man who had lectured and consulted everywhere, who stood up virtually single-handedly and at great potential cost to his career against the loyalty oaths that had been imposed upon all grant applicants by the Public Health Service during the McCarthy era. He very publicly boycotted the NIH, refusing to accept scientists funded by the Public Health Service into his laboratory, and continued to do so until, in his version of events at least, the government backed down and rescinded the requirement several years later. As a boy, I remember the day he came home and opened a bottle of champagne for us to celebrate the victory. His gods were principled behavior and honesty, his commanding ethic as a scientist... to let the data speak for itself. As far as I know, he never deviated from that principle in his scientific work.

He had published close to five hundred scientific papers from his laboratory, in collaboration with colleagues from all over the world. He had co-authored three editions of a weighty textbook, *Experimental Immunochemistry*, the "bible" of its time in the field, as well as other technical books that I could hardly understand a word of, even given my training in molecular biology. And here he was now, confusing deductions with reimbursements, asking me whose house it was when he came to visit me; assuring me with some satisfaction that he had a special relationship with the telephone company that allowed him to write out deposit slips to them rather than checks when paying his phone bills, and being so convincing and endearing that for a moment he almost had me believing it; recounting on occasion how he had lived with the Pygmies in Africa for a time and how, when he arrived in their village, he found that they were "very happy" to see him and that they had already read all his scientific papers and books. The image of small people looking up to him and honoring him did not escape notice. When I asked him where that was in Africa, he said, "South America." And so it went. He wandered. He became incontinent. He didn't understand any more about his own work. He became more and more vague about who his friends were.

I treasured our time together, no matter what was happening as the curtain of dementia descended on his memory and his knowing of where he was and what was happening to him. We would sit together holding hands, sometimes for hours. He could sit for a long time. It was as if we were meditating together. He was present in his way and I in mine. Most importantly, we were together. Our time together was precious, painful, exasperating.

He did have his moments. One day, sitting in the garden, facing a tall stockade fence behind which rose a telephone pole against a backdrop of bushes and sky, with a lone wire coming to it and nothing going out (it must have descended into the ground along the back of the pole), at one point he declared, out of nowhere, "That really is the end of the line."

It was so true. I flashed to what the photograph would look like of the two of us sitting on the bench, from behind, with the telephone pole and its lone wire in front of us, against the sky. It could have been called "the end of the line." For him, it was.

Another time, commenting on the coming and going of the ambulances he could see from his window at the assisted living center, he observed: "When you die, they kick you out."

I came to feel more and more the ebbing of his faculties of mind and body, and for some time, he did too, and railed against it, until even that dissolved. But he never did not know who his wife was or who his children or grandchildren were. He could identify us to the end by voice alone on the telephone. I would call up and say, "Hi, Dad," and he would instantly know who it was, that it was me and not one of my two brothers, whose voices are a lot like mine. His affectionate greeting, "Hi, Jonny darling," killed me with poignancy, and gratitude, and sadness.

On the day that he died, I had been holding him in my arms for some hours, singing his favorite songs from Gilbert and Sullivan to him, songs that he had sung to me as a baby, but making up new words now and again to bathe him in messages about how much he was loved, how much he lived in the love of his family, and how it was now all right for him to go. Interspersed with these, I had been chanting all the chants I had learned over the years from the various traditions I had practiced in, including the Heart Sutra in both English and Korean, then falling into long stretches of silence. It felt right, somehow, to be intoning "form does not differ from emptiness, emptiness does not differ from form," with tears streaming down my face. Through it all, especially in the long silences, I was acutely aware of his breathing, so tentative and irregular, as well as my own. Then there came, at one moment, after many hours, an exhalation that hung suspended. It was not followed by an in-breath. I held him for a long time, sobbing.

Much was revealed to me about what I was taking so for granted through the eight long years in which my father was losing his mind. Increasingly he was out of touch with what had just transpired even a few moments before. He was present, but it was a bewildered, befuddled presence. He was unaware of the context of things. He was not oriented in an inclusive awareness that held a feeling for the past and the future. He was often stymied in trying to convey concepts he clearly had but were somehow just out of reach of his mind and his tongue. He would be talking about specific things, but would have to resort out of frustration to using the word "substance" or "material," which he had used a lot in his scientific vocabulary, to invoke what he was talking about, and we just couldn't understand, it was all so vague. Relationships outside his immediate family became more and more blurry over time. But his emotions were still intact. After a horrific and horrifying period of intense frustration and anger brought on by his plight and his inability to do anything about it, despite all his attempts to hold on to his life and his lab and his world, he gradually became more gentle and more overtly loving. He also became increasingly lonely, more and more isolated in his own world. He was happy for any attention. He loved attention. That had always been a salient part of his character, no matter how much the world acknowledged his numerous accomplishments. But even toward the end, it still had to be respectful attention, and engaging of his interests. He could tell the difference if someone was just going through the motions, humoring him, or being condescending.

My father's illness showed me how important it is to make use of the full spectrum of our mental capacities while we have them and are in a position to stop taking them for granted. I learned how important it is to develop those capacities in the service of discerning the actuality of things, not getting seduced by mere appearance and mistaking it for reality. That never happened to my father as a scientist, but like all of us, he was not immune to its happening in other aspects of his life.

Ultimately, we all need to know, and unless we are afflicted with Alzheimer's or some other form of dementia, we all do know our location in time and space in every moment (even if it is to know that we are lost). And we all need to know and be in touch with the relative sense of knowing who each of us is, as well as where (here) and when (now), and to be able to situate ourselves within a stream of befores and afters, and of where we were when.

In ways we do not yet understand, our nervous system takes care of these orienting functions for us, and does a remarkable job of it across the life span. But we would do well to keep in mind that it is a quality of mind that itself is impermanent, not guaranteed, and easily taken for granted. In cultivating mindfulness, we are making maximal use of it while we have the chance.

The loss of this basic orienting function is chillingly evoked in the opening scene of Alan Lightman's novel *The Diagnosis*, in which, somewhere between suburban Alewife station and his destination in downtown Boston, a businessman commuter simply and inexplicably forgets who he is and where he is going. The surreal nightmare of losing one's purpose and orientation ("Where am I going this morning, all dressed up for work? Oh yes. To the office, course, like all these other people on the train. But where do I work, and what is it that actually I do?") leads all of a sudden to immersion in a dreamlike state in which everything is vaguely familiar and yet not. It rapidly turns into a living nightmare.

We live on the cusp of such boundaries at all times. Yet somehow, our orienting system is so robust that we are saved from the pathology of the nightmare, at least on the conventional level. But "Who am I?" and "Where am I going?" are deep questions, Zen koans* really, and the suggestion is that we would benefit deeply from asking them of ourselves on a regular basis, as a meditation practice, rather than simply taking who we are and what we do for granted, especially if we think we know and are not so inclined to ask such questions and peel back the veil of appearance and the stories we tell ourselves that may be covering over the deep structure and multiple dimensions and textures of our actual lives. For none of us ever know how long we can count on having these capacities at our disposal, or how long we actually have to continue living and learning and growing into the fullness of ourselves.

For my father, what remained when his memory and understanding were almost entirely gone was the love of his family, the deep bonds with his many wonderful friends, colleagues, and students around the globe, and what he had done and given to and loved in the world. These are our most human threads of connection. But they too

---

* A koan is a Zen teaching device, like a puzzle in the form of a question or statement or dialogue one attempts to hold in mind during meditation and understand and respond to without responding with the discursive thinking mind, since no response coming out of thought will be authentic and adequate to the circumstances of the moment. An example would be "Who am I?" or "Does a dog have Buddha nature?" or "What is Buddha?" Almost any life circumstance could be seen as a koan. You could think of it as "What is this?" or even, "What now?" In every moment, the response might be different. The only requirement is that it be authentic and appropriate, and not come out of dualistic thinking. Responses can be non-verbal.

are evanescent and transient, best recognized, cultivated, and enjoyed while we have the chance.

For any of us, perhaps our greatest potential regret may be that of not seizing the moment and honoring it for what it is when it is here, especially in regard to our relationships with people and with nature. Perhaps that is the ultimate orientation, both within space and time, and simultaneously beyond space and time: a seamless continuity of knowing what is, directly, non-conceptually, experientially. And loving it.

Orthogonal Reality—Rotating in Consciousness

As a rule, we humans have been admirable explorers and inhabitants of conventional reality, the world "out there" defined and modulated by our five classical senses. We have made ourselves at home within that world, and have learned to shape it to our needs and desires over the brief course of human history. We understand cause and effect in the physical world, at least the Newtonian physical world, to an ever-increasing degree due to the efforts of science, and that understanding is continuing to deepen with ongoing discoveries.

And yet even within science, looking at the edges, it is not so clear that we comprehend underlying reality, which seems disturbingly statistical, unpredictable, and mysterious, as per the causes and timing of a particular radioactive decay event in the nucleus of a radioactive atom; or whether the universe is finite or not, or even only one of an infinite number of universes within various multiverses; or whether time even exists; or what happens in the heart of a black hole; or why the vacuum has so much energy; or the question of whether space is nothing or something.

Nevertheless, in the conventional everyday reality of lived experience, as noted earlier, we have a body, we are born, we live out our lives and we die. For the most part, we dwell mostly accepting the appearance of things and create quasi-comfortable explanations for ourselves about how things are and why they are that way. And all the while, our senses can lull us to sleep, especially if we are coasting on habit, not really in touch from moment to moment, so caught up are we in thinking and doing, and thus somewhat removed from the domain of being, from sentience, even though it is closer than close at all moments.

I say to Myla as a young person passes by us in the street: "He has such a nice face." To which she responds: "Yes, if you don't see the lack of affect in it."

It is all a matter of what we are willing to see or reflexively ignore, how reflexively we are willing to berth our momentary perceptions at the dock of the habitually inattentive, secured by stout lines of really-not-looking-but-pretending-to-yourself-that-you-are rope.

In the world of this conventional reality, we do the best we can. We earn a living, we put food on the table, we love our children and care for our parents, do our work and whatever else we need to do to maintain our forward momentum through life and perhaps learn to *dance*, as Zorba did, even in the face of the poignant existential realities of the human condition: stress, pain, illness, old age, and death, Zorba's "full catastrophe." All the while, we are immersed in a stream of thoughts whose origins and content are frequently unclear to us and which can be obsessive, repetitive, inaccurate, disturbingly unrelenting and toxic, all of which both color the present moment and shield it from us. Moreover, we are frequently hijacked by emotions we cannot control and that can cause great harm to ourselves and to others, or are the result of earlier harm or perceived harm. These also prevent us from seeing with any clarity, even though our eyes are open.

Unpleasant moments are bewildering and disconcerting. So they are apt to be written off as aberrations or impediments to the ever-hoped-for happiness we are seeking and the story we build around it. Such moments get papered over by persistent inattention, and are soon forgotten. Alternatively, we might build an equally tenacious unpleasant story around our failures, our inadequacies, and our misdeeds to explain why we cannot transcend our limitations and our karma, and then, in thinking that it is all true, forget that it is just one more story we are telling ourselves, and cling desperately to it as if our very identity, our very survival, and all hope were unquestionably bound to it.

What we also forget is that the conventional consensus reality we call the human condition is itself inexorably and strongly *conditioned* in the Pavlovian sense.

As a result of this lifelong conditioning, we are not really as "free" as we think when we think we are free to do whatever we want, which may mean that we are totally at the mercy of our mind's habitual grasping and pushing away. We do not even perceive our own potential for freedom in the sense that Einstein or the Buddha spoke of it. Why? Because we forget or do not know that we do not have to be perpetually caught up in reactions to events, in our often unconscious decisions to do this or that, relate in this or that way, see things this way or that way, avoid this or that, forget this or that, including that all this conditioning adds up to the appearance of a life, but often one that remains disturbingly superficial and unsatisfying, with a lingering sense that there must be something more, some deeper meaning, some possibility for being comfortable in one's own skin, independent of conditions, whether things are momentarily "good" or "bad," "pleasant" or "unpleasant."

We feel such discomfort, such disappointment, such discontentment and realize at times that it may be all-pervasive, a kind of silent background radiation of dissatisfaction in us all that, as a rule, we don't talk about. Usually it is unilluminating, just oppressive. Hmmm... sounds a lot like dukkha, dukkha, and more dukkha (See Book 1, *Meditation Is Not What You Think*, Part 2).

But, when we look into what that dis-affection, that background unsatisfactoriness actually is, when we are drawn to actually question and look into "Who is suffering?" in this moment, we are undertaking an exploration of another dimension of reality altogether—one that offers unrecognized but ever-available freedom from the confining prison of the conventional thought world, even as we pay it its due and continue to recognize its now more limited and potentially less limiting existence. Our very interest in freedom from suffering and in not causing suffering unnecessarily and unwittingly becomes a doorway into realizing a new dimension in being and an expanded way of living, based on the primacy of relationality and interconnectedness.

The process feels like nothing other than an awakening from a consensus trance, a dream world, and thus all of a sudden acquiring multiple degrees of freedom, many more options for seeing and responding and for meeting wholeheartedly and with mindfulness whatever situations we find ourselves in, that before we might have just reacted to out of deeply embedded and conditioned habits. It is akin to the transition from a two-dimensional "flatland" into a third spatial dimension, at right angles (orthogonal) to the other two. Everything opens up, even though the two "old" dimensions are the same as they always were. But they are now less confining because we have added or discovered that third dimension.

Just by asking, for instance, "Who is suffering?" "Who doesn't want what is happening to be happening?" "Who is frightened?" "Who is thinking?" "Who is feeling insecure, or unwanted, or lost?" or "What am I?" we are initiating nothing less than a rotation in consciousness into another "dimension," orthogonal to conventional reality, and thus, able to pertain at the same time as the more conventional ones because you have simply "added more space," in fact a whole new dimension. Nothing needs to change. It's just that your world immediately becomes a lot bigger, and more real. Everything old looks different because it is now being seen in a new light—an awareness that is no longer confined by the more limited and limiting conventional dimensionality and mind-set.

As for change, it is always happening anyway. Often we are impeding natural change and growth through our own efforts to force things to be a certain way, which actually *contracts* the reality, keeps us locked in the conditioned mind and our conditioned views by collapsing those other up to now hidden dimensions and options that, when tapped into, offer us new degrees of freedom in both our inner and outer landscapes.

When you have an experience of rotating in consciousness so that your world *does* all of a sudden feel bigger and more real, you are catching a glimpse of what Buddhists refer to as absolute or ultimate reality, a dimensionality that is beyond conditioning but that is capable of recognizing conditioning as it arises. It is awareness itself, the knowing capacity of mind itself, beyond a knower and what is known, just knowing. And interestingly, it is already here, and already yours.

When we reside in awareness, we are resting in what we might call an *orthogonal reality* that is more fundamental than conventional reality, and every bit as real. Both pertain moment by moment, and both demand their due if we are to inhabit and embody the full scope of our humanness, our true nature as sentient beings.

When we inhabit this orthogonal dimension or dimensions, the problems of the conventional reality are seen from a different perspective, more spacious than that of a small-minded self-interest. The situations we face can thus admit possibilities of freedom, resolution, acceptance, creativity, compassion, and wisdom that were literally inconceivable—unable to arise and sustain—within the conventional mind set.

This expanded universe of freedom is the promise of mindfulness both in our individual lives and in the world. In the world, it can involve a rotation in consciousness on the part of many people in a relatively short time. Such a shift can immediately reveal the nature of a difficult situation in a new light, in all its complexity and its simplicity, with added dimensions and degrees of freedom and possibility...for new insight, for wise action, and for healing. That is what an orthogonal perspective offers. That is what mindfulness offers... insight into what is most fundamental and most important, and most easily forgotten or lost. The conventional reality is not "wrong." It is merely incomplete. And therein lies the source of both our suffering and our liberation from suffering.

We are not strangers to orthogonal shifts. An authentic apology, for instance, as Aaron Lazare deftly demonstrated in *On Apology*, can instantly dissolve long-standing rancor, resentment, humiliation, guilt, and shame in both parties, and lead to almost instantaneous healing, forgiveness, expressions of love, and caring, among both individual people, and even between nations. What seemed highly improbable if not totally impossible the moment before can and does actually happen. What one thought was a "forbidden transition" in oneself is discovered to not only be not forbidden, but profoundly possible, where the moment before, it was inconceivable. The condition of happiness following the apology is orthogonal to the condition of suffering before the apology. It was present all the time as a potential, as possible, but it required a rotation within the mindscape and heartscape in order to manifest as real. And in undergoing that transition, old wounds are healed, old hurts forgiven, and new understandings, reconciliations, and spaciousness of heart and mind seemingly magically emerge.

Orthogonal Institutions

If individuals can rotate in consciousness, so can institutions, and even nations. After all, we now have very different views of slavery than those widely held in this country two hundred years ago; we have very different views about gender and women's rights, and what constitutes harassment; we no longer routinely keep a cancer diagnosis from patients so as not to upset them, as happened in medicine for decades. These all involved collective rotations in consciousness, in how we see things and what we understand to be of primary importance, and then how we embody that understanding in the world—how we actually act, including the laws we enact or don't. How deeply these realizations make their way into law is another matter altogether, and often victims continue to be victimized by the powerful who control and regulate those laws, with little practical recourse. Any enduring changes in the social order usually reflect strong activism on someone's part, often on the part of large numbers of people over many decades, demanding change from either the inside or the outside, exhibiting moral outrage, speaking truths that may be unpleasant to hear, sometimes even dying for their cause. The inertia and vested interests in maintaining the status quo in any situation or institution are not likely to either initiate or sustain the motive force behind an orthogonal rotation in perspective. Nevertheless, when minds change, and vision changes, and people taste new possibilities for healing past wrongs or correcting fundamentally problematic situations, for making democracy more democratic, for insuring equal opportunity and basic human rights, usually interesting things happen that were previously thought to be impossible, or were never thought of at all. As a rule, our society and our institutions are the better for it because these rotations in consciousness tend to move us in the direction of a more refined embodiment and actualization of humane values: of freedom for each and every person to pursue his or her virtually infinite and always unknown potential; and to live in peace and experience well-being, free potentially from inner and outer harm.

To my mind, an orthogonal institution would be one that had rotated in consciousness to some degree and could thus exist, as noted in the last chapter, in the same space, but with a larger dimensionality, and at the same time as more conventional elements of the institution, or exist on its own within the larger conventional reality and thus redefine and expand its own sense of purpose and perhaps larger and unimagined but imaginable possibilities.

In that sense, as an individual, bringing a sustained openhearted awareness to your work or your family can make your work or your family functionally orthogonal to the conventional mind set and coordinate system within which things usually tend to operate. It brings the inner and outer landscapes together into one seamless, undivided whole, one that allows for all our intelligences to be present simultaneously, and for us to thus let our doing, whatever it is, come out of our being, and thus, out of our innate wisdom and potential for wise and compassionate action, even in the face of inward or outward conflict, or groups holding widely divergent and polarized views. Here too, undreamed of possibilities abound for inclusivity and for win-win options that reflect one's commitment to a greater wisdom—yet take courage and deep vision to enact.

The Stress Reduction Clinic, and MBSR (mindfulness-based stress reduction) more generally, grounded as they are in mindfulness, have always functioned by design and intention from the very beginning as an orthogonal institution*, aimed at bringing the methods and perspectives of mindfulness and of mindfulness-based mind/body approaches to health and healing into the mainstream of medicine. Just bringing the worlds of meditation and medicine together in 1979, to say nothing of including yoga, was, you might say, something of a stretch, an interpenetration of perspectives that ordinarily had virtually nothing to do with each other. From the point of view of the medicine of that time, meditation might have easily been seen as flaky, unscientific, and of no practical value or even, potentially, of negative value—as I sometimes quipped, "the Visigoths are at the gates, about to tear down the hard-won edifices of scientific-based medicine and health care, and maybe even the very citadel of Western

---

* I came up with the term "orthogonal institution" in 1969—in the middle of the Vietnam War and the Cold War, as a graduate student at MIT and a co-founder of its Science Action Coordination Committee (SACC) to try to get across to the community (which tends to be familiar with words such as *orthogonal*) why the institution as a whole needed to take responsibility for the uses and abuses of science in terms of developing increasingly sophisticated technologies for killing people by designing delivery systems for weapons of mass destruction, exceedingly well-incentivized by grant money from the Department of Defense. It was an attempt to catalyze a "rotation in consciousness" on the part of the institution as a whole, not just MIT, but all scientific institutions, in relationship to war-related research so they might take a fresh look at the social and political consequences of their intellectual and scholarly pursuits. As students, we were often told that we should do something constructive with our education rather than just "destroying" venerable existing institutions, which of course was never our objective. But ten years later, MBSR was an attempt on my part to ultimately do just that, i.e. create an orthogonal institution within medicine and health care at the University of Massachusetts Medical Center, and see whether it might not have a transformative effect on how medicine was practiced, including engaging people with chronic medical problems to participate in their own trajectory toward greater levels of well-being and health through fairly rigorous training in mindfulness as a complement to whatever their doctors were able to do for them. To the degree that MBSR has contributed to a far-greater credence in (and evidence for) the value of such an approach, it has in fact served that orthogonal function fairly effectively over the past forty years, and has contributed to transforming the mind-set and practices of medicine itself.

Civilization itself." Yet the orthogonal perspective inherent in MBSR and in mindfulness allowed them to coexist with medicine in the early years in a way that slowly revealed how much they had in common (let's not forget that *medicine* and *meditation* obviously share the same etymological root) and how much they could serve each other and augment in profound ways what could be offered to a wide range of patients with chronic conditions of all kinds in terms of participating in tangible and meaningful ways in their own health and health care, and well-being.

From the outside, the Stress Reduction Clinic looked like any other clinic in the hospital. It had a name, a location, and official signs in the corridors to get you there. It was (and is) part of the Department of Medicine. It had a patient brochure and billing procedures. As it grew, it came to have a director and an associate director, an administrator, a staff of receptionists and instructors. When it started out, we used borrowed offices, even closets, and various spaces nobody wanted. For a long time, we used the Faculty Conference Room and then the Rare Book Room in the medical school library as our classroom space. Our lack of designated space for our clinic didn't really matter. Over time, we came to have lovely office space and a welcoming reception area, a great classroom, and plenty of smaller rooms in which to hold private interviews with the patients who were referred to us, and ultimately, our own building. But through all these changes, the clinic has continued to function like any other clinic. It billed like a clinic, paid its employees like a clinic, everybody in the medical center called it a clinic, and doctors referred their patients to it, just as they did to other clinics.

Yet, whether you walked into the reception area for a scheduled appointment, or into an interview room for a private individual assessment, or into the classroom for a class, in a very real way you were walking into another reality, even as you were still very much in the conventional one. Although you might not have known it fully at the time, your world was being invited to rotate in consciousness, to expand to include unsuspected dimensions of possibility. For aside from being a clinic in the hospital, the Stress Reduction Clinic was and is, to this day, also another planet, in an orthogonal universe. The universe of mindfulness and heartfulness, the universe of wholeness, of embodied wakefulness.

Right from the start, people tended to feel that something was different. For the staff, it was nothing particularly special, just an intentional and commonsensical commitment to be as mindful as possible, to be present for people, to listen, to be kind, to be explicit about what could be described and explicit about what couldn't be, to embody what any hospital would want its employees to embody, openhearted presence—not in theory, but in actual day-to-day and moment-to-moment practice. And while being nothing special, it was and is to this day extremely special.

From the very beginning, the primary intention of those of us working in the MBSR clinic, whatever our official job description, was to adhere as best we could to Hippocratic principles, to see everyone who was referred to us first as human beings rather than as patients, intrinsically capable of limitless growing and learning. It was axiomatic that we bring mindfulness to our work, and pay attention to all aspects of it in a sustained, openhearted, empathic way; that we work as best we were able in any moment to be fully present, and without unacknowledged and unexamined agendas that might interfere with rather than enhance our encounters with the patients and our efforts to engage them in meaningful ways regarding the various meditation practices and their potential power to influence their lives if they gave their practice a serious chance over the eight weeks of the program.

And it was axiomatic that we not try to sell anything to anybody, leaving the decision to the patients as to whether or not to enroll in the program. But when they came in to be interviewed, we endeavored to meet them as openheartedly as we could, and made a point of listening with undivided attention to their recounting of what brought them to the clinic, for listening deeply is a defining quality of mindfulness meditation. Then, when it seemed right, we described for them what they could expect if they took the program, not in terms of promised outcomes, but as a process, and an adventure of sorts, and why relatively intensive training in mindfulness meditation might have some relevance to their particular situation, if we thought it did.

From the very beginning, we presented MBSR as a major challenge, and made it very clear that it was a huge lifestyle change just to take the program, as it involved committing to coming to class once a week for eight weeks, plus participating in an all-day silent retreat on the weekend in the sixth week, plus daily meditation practice using audio devices, first tapes, then CDs, then digital apps for guidance for at least forty-five minutes a day, six days per week. I often found myself saying that you didn't have to *like* practicing the meditation for homework in this disciplined way; you just had to do it, whether you felt like it or not, whether you liked it or not, suspending judgment as best you could along the way. Then, at the end of the eight weeks of the program, you could let us know whether it was beneficial or not (although I sometimes used much more colorful language in making this point). But in between, the contract was that you would just keep practicing and coming to class, whether on any given day you felt good about the practice or hated it. You still had to do it.

I also found myself saying on occasion that just as firefighters sometimes have to start a fire to put out a larger fire, so they might find it stressful just to take the stress reduction program; and that, no matter how much we described the meditation practices to them in advance, they would not really have any idea what they were getting themselves into until they actually started practicing. I also tended to tell people that from our perspective, there was more right with them than wrong with them, no matter what was wrong, no matter what diagnosis or diagnoses they had been given, or the magnitude and poignancy of the full catastrophe in their lives. The basic invitation was that working together, we were going to pour energy into what was right with them over a period of eight weeks, let their doctor and the rest of their medical team, if necessary, take care of what was wrong—and just see what would happen. At the close of these intake interviews, the patients decided for themselves whether it was something they wanted to engage in or not.

This meant that no one was in the classroom under duress. You had to want to be there to join. People were continually voting with their feet. For the most part, they hadn't been met in quite that way before by the health care system, with that level of matter-of-fact but openhearted presence, and with an unwavering regard for their potential to tap deep interior resources of mind and body to deal with whatever aspect of the full catastrophe was bringing each of them to the clinic.

And for the most part, people felt it, then, and do to this day. They may not know what it is at first, but most of us feel better when we are seen and heard and met with authentic presence and regard, without condescension or contrived intimacy. We feel good when we are treated as capable, when we are related to as if we have the capacity to actually undertake the hardest work in the world, when a lot is being asked of us, but in ways that build on our own intrinsic capacities and intelligences. Well over 26,000 people have taken the MBSR program at UMass and scores of thousands in MBSR programs across the country and around the world.

Among ourselves we joked about how at times it felt as if we could have just as well gone by the name Mindlessness-Based Stress Production Clinic, given the pace, intensity, and demands of the work environment in which we were embedded and the pressures intrinsic to serving a continual stream of people who are suffering, coupled with the endless tasks and projects needing to get done for things to work well, just as in any other job or work environment. But the commitment among the teachers and staff to see work itself as practice, to bring mindfulness into all aspects of it and not just into the classroom, nourished us and gave us infinite and humbling opportunities to see and marvel at how mindless and attached we could sometimes be. Seeing work itself as practice encouraged us to recommit over and over again to rotating in awareness, to embodying mindfulness and non-attachment, to being fully present with what is, whatever that looked like in any moment or on any given day, and to face whatever it called for us to deal with in that moment, leavened with a healthy dose of humor.

You could call such an orientation *the Tao of Work*. Nothing could be more challenging, or more satisfying. And ultimately, since it is all based on non-doing, it actually is nothing, and we don't have to do anything for it to flourish, or make a big deal of it either. We do nothing, yet, as in the Way of the Tao, nothing is left undone. That's the overriding attitude and perspective. In addition, of course, it also takes a huge amount of work and continually attempting to find a dynamical moment-by-moment balance between all the doing and the non-doing. For, ironically, as people engaged in the work of MBSR have all discovered, it takes a lot of doing to nurture appropriate conditions to further non-doing, and to respond to the various demands and challenges of running a stress reduction clinic in a busy medical environment, especially one that may not understand the benefits of orthogonality.

It is also ironic that awareness, intentionality, and kindness may still be sadly undernourished in many hospital settings, especially since these qualities are what hospitals are ostensibly all about. The very word "hospital" betokens hospitality, an honored greeting, a true receiving. But somehow it is still all too easy within hospitals and the stream of medical care, although nobody *intends* for it to happen, to get lost, to not be fully met or heard or seen, and perhaps to not be followed to the point of completion and personal satisfaction. The people within the system can all be terrific, yet the system can nevertheless fail many of its patients.

In so many ways, the world is crying out for orthogonal institutions that could be co-extensive with existent ones or for brand-new stand-alones, orthogonal in the larger world. They do exist...anywhere and everywhere people embody the principles of caring for the greater good, inquire deeply as to what that might entail, and then take care of what needs taking care of, inwardly and outwardly—since in the end, any separation of inner and outer is merely a conventional convenience.

A Study in Healing
and the Mind

Picture this: A person with the skin disease psoriasis, standing practically naked in a cylindrical lightbox lined with vertical eight-foot-long ultraviolet lightbulbs that form a complete enclosure. Her eyes are shielded by dark goggles to protect the corneas from UV damage, plus she is wearing a pillowcase over her head to protect her face. (Her nipples are also shielded, as are the genitals in men.) Fans whir, circulating stale basement-office air in the bowels of the medical center. When the lights come on, bathing not just the lightbox and the patient inside it, but, because the top is open, the entire room with an eerie violet glow, their intensity is ferocious, irradiating every surface of the body that is exposed with specifically chosen and particularly potent wavelengths of ultraviolet light.

The treatment is known as phototherapy. In order to prevent the skin from burning, the person comes for treatment three times a week for many weeks, and the length of exposure is gradually increased, from about thirty seconds at the beginning to maybe ten to fifteen minutes after a few weeks, depending on the patient's skin type, fair skin being of course more prone to burning. Over time, the raised, red, inflamed patches of skin, which in severe cases cover large parts of the body, begin to flatten and change color, looking more and more like the person's normal skin. When the treatment is complete, the skin looks entirely normal and clear. There are no more scaly patches.

The treatment is not a cure, however. The unsightly patches can return. Recurrent episodes are often triggered by psychological stress.

Little is known about the genetic predisposition, the primary causes, or the molecular biology of the disease. It is definitely an uncontrolled cell proliferation in the epidermal layer of the skin, but it is not cancer. The rapidly growing cells do not invade other tissues, nor does the disease result in ill health or death. It is, however, disfiguring in some cases, and can be psychologically debilitating. It carries whatever social onus and vulnerability accompanies having skin that looks different and not being able to hide it completely. It can feel like having the plague. The novelist John Updike captured the poignancy of this affliction as only a writer of his talent who knew it from the inside could:

Oct. 31. I have long been a potter, a bachelor, and a leper. Leprosy is not exactly what I have, but what in the Bible is called leprosy was probably this thing, which has a twisty Greek name it pains me to write. The form of the disease is as follows: spots, plaques, and avalanches of excess skin, manufactured by the dermis through some trifling but persistent error in its metabolic instructions, expand and slowly migrate across the body like lichen on a tombstone. I am silvery, scaly. Puddles of flakes form wherever I rest my flesh. Each morning I vacuum my bed. My torture is skin deep: There is no pain, not even itching; we lepers live a long time, and are ironically healthy in other respects. Lusty, though we are loathsome to love. Keen-sighted, though we hate to look upon ourselves. The name of the disease, spiritually speaking, is Humiliation.

Nov. 1. The doctor whistles when I take off my clothes. "Quite a case."...The floor of his office, I notice, is sprinkled with flakes. There are other lepers. At last, I am not alone... As I drag my clothes on, a shower of silver falls to the floor. He calls it, professionally, "scale." I call it, inwardly, filth.

JOHN UPDIKE, "From the Journal of a Leper," *New Yorker*, 1976

I learned about psoriasis and phototherapy one day at a Department of Medicine retreat in the early 1980s. I happened to sit down for lunch with a young, cheerful-looking man who as it turned out was the chief of dermatology, Dr. Jeff Bernhard. We got to talking, and when he found out I ran the department's stress reduction clinic and that we taught Buddhist meditative practices to the patients (albeit "without the Buddhism," as I sometimes put it), he asked me if I knew the book *Zen Mind, Beginner's Mind*, by Shunryu Suzuki.

I was amazed just to hear that he had read it and further amazed that he loved it. So we fell to talking about meditation and Zen, and about how we (the Department of Medicine) were offering the rudiments and what we hoped was the essence of just such training and practices as Suzuki was talking about (modified of course for the secular hospital setting in an entirely different culture) to our patients. I saw the lightbulb go off in his head as he asked me if I thought we could train his psoriasis patients undergoing treatment in the phototherapy clinic to relax while they were in the lightbox.

He then described the disease and its treatment pretty much the way I have just done. He also explained that undergoing phototherapy was a very stressful experience for his patients for a number of reasons. First, the patients had to come to the hospital three times a week for very short treatments, so short that finding a parking place could take longer than the treatments themselves. Then the patient had to undress and cover his or her body with oil, a messy proposition in its own right, then put on the black goggles and the pillowcase, and stand naked in the confining space of the lightbox in the heat and the stale air, with the oppressive intensity of the lights roasting the skin, with motor noises filling the air; then shower to get off the oil or leave it on, as many did, get dressed, and get to their car. Treatments took place only during the day, so having to do this three times a week for up to three months was a real inconvenience and a major disruption of one's daily life and routine, especially if the patient had a job. Plus, they were unable to read magazines or distract themselves in the usual ways patients do when they are undergoing treatment. The whole thing had a kind of undignified and burdensome aura to it.

Was there any way, Jeff asked, that what we were doing with our patients in the Stress Reduction Clinic might help his phototherapy patients to be more relaxed and deal with the stress of their treatments in a better way? He was concerned because many of his patients stopped coming regularly even before their skin cleared, and others just dropped out because the treatments were so disruptive, and perhaps, also because, since the disease was not life-threatening, the incentive to undergo the extensive course of treatment wasn't always great. It was usually for cosmetic reasons. Moreover, the effect of the treatment was only temporary, not being a permanent cure.

Could meditation, Jeff wanted to know, make the whole experience of phototherapy more pleasant for his patients and increase their motivation for staying with the treatment protocol?

As he was saying this and I was picturing what he was describing in my mind, lightbulbs (no pun intended) were starting to go off in my own head. Yes, I replied. We could certainly teach his patients effective methods to relax while they were in the lightbox, and for dealing with the unpleasant aspects of the treatment. It seemed to be a perfect situation for guiding them in the practice of standing meditation, since they had to be standing in the lightbox anyway. That could include breathing meditation, hearing meditation, feeling-the-light-on-the-skin meditation, and watching-the-mind-get-stressed-out meditation, in a word, a full spectrum of mindfulness practices tailored to their moment-to-moment experience in the lightbox. And, I said, I had no doubt that at least some of his patients would be more relaxed as a result, and might actually enjoy their treatments more because they would be participating actively in the treatment and engaging their own powers of attention, thereby possibly neutralizing some of the more onerous features that would cause high dropout rates.

But, I continued, we could do something even more adventurous. It struck me that the phototherapy paradigm was perfect for studying the important question of whether and how the mind might influence healing; in this case, a healing process that we could actually see unfolding and photograph and track over time. Why not train his psoriasis patients in these mindfulness-based practices as part of a small clinical trial to see whether we could detect effects of the mind itself on the rate of skin clearing? We could randomize potential subjects into two groups. In one, the patients would meditate while they were standing in the lightbox, guided by an audiotape (this was the only audio technology available back in the 1980s) designed specifically for their situation. In the other group, the patients would get the light treatments in the usual way, without the meditation instructions. And, just to maximize the chance of finding something, I proposed that we include a visualization about the skin healing in response to the light as part of the meditation in the later stages of treatment, when the sessions run longer and there would be more time to hear such instructions.

We went ahead and set up a pilot study along these lines, just to see what would happen. What we found was that the meditators' skin cleared on average much more rapidly than in the case of the non-meditators. With this encouraging result under our belt, we then set out to repeat the study to convince ourselves that it was not a fluke, and to do it with more patients and with a more rigorous study protocol, in which we used several different methods to rate the patients' skin status over time, including regularly photographing their most prominent lesions and having two dermatologists rate the photographs independently, without knowing which group the patients were in, nor who they were.

Again, we found that the meditators healed faster than the non-meditators and this time we were able to say something about how much faster. It turned out that the statistics were showing that the meditators were clearing almost four times as rapidly as the non-meditators.*

While this study was under way, the well-known journalist, Bill Moyers was filming in the Stress Reduction Clinic for a PBS television special that would be called *Healing and the Mind*. It was frustrating to have a study in progress that addressed this very question yet be unable to speak of it, because until enough patients were recruited into the study and completed the protocol, we didn't want any publicity about it, which might have influenced the outcome and also made it more difficult to get our results published. What's more, we were waiting to look at the data and analyze the results until we had a large enough number of participants to make it sensible to go ahead, so we had no idea what kind of results we were getting, if any. By the time we had reached the point where we had enough patients in the study to begin the data analysis, the filming for the program had already taken place.

Once the study was published, a number of years later, we were able to talk about it publicly and discuss what our results might imply about the possible effects of the mind on the healing process, or at least, one healing process.

Because the meditators healed so much more rapidly than the control group, professional audiences frequently ask, "What is on that tape?" as if there must be something especially magical that would produce such a dramatic result. But what is on the tape is very ordinary, just mindfulness instructions and the visualization, and short stretches of silence in between. I sometimes quip that nothing is on the tape, just silence, and instructions on how to be in the silence

---

* Kabat-Zinn, J., Wheeler, E., Light, T., Skillings, A., Scharf, M., Cropley, T. G., Hosmer, D., and Bernhard, J. "Influence of a mindfulness-based stress reduction intervention on rates of skin clearing in patients with moderate to severe psoriasis undergoing phototherapy (UVB) and photochemotherapy (PUVA)." *Psychosomatic Medicine* 60 (1998): 625–632.

and make use of it. That is true in spirit, less so practically speaking, because in somewhat under fifteen minutes under those conditions (no class, no instructor, no homework, and thus very different from MBSR), you need a good deal of spoken instruction to cover the various aspects of the meditation practice.

Yet the guidance on the tape was really all about cultivating a deep inner silence and openness beneath even the instructions, in which one could give oneself over with full attention, with full presence of mind and body to the moments of standing there in the lightbox and experiencing the light itself, along with the intention that it do its work of helping the skin to clear.

Since both the disease and the treatment concerned the skin, it was natural that the meditation instructions focused on cultivating a heightened and sustained awareness of the envelope of the body that is the skin, imagining it "breathing," and feeling all the sensations associated with exposure to the light, such as intense heat, and the sensation of the air, blown by the fans, moving across the skin and around the body.

While certainly in need of replication and much more detailed research into the possible mechanisms by which the healing would be taking place, our study points to a potential for intentional healing that could be important. We hope that other dermatologists will attempt to replicate our findings and extend them well beyond what we were able to do, especially with the new molecular technologies available in this era.

I like to think of the result we obtained in this study as reflecting a potential inherent in all of us, one we have seen expressed over and over again in different ways in the Stress Reduction Clinic when our patients are invited and encouraged to become active participants in their own medical treatment and health care.*

Whether alone in the lightbox, or meditating as a participant in an MBSR program with other people, I see a medical patient's active involvement in his or her own health care as an example of what

---

* Margaret Donald's letter to me in the Foreword is an example of this.

might be called *participatory medicine*,* where the doctor has her or his role in the treatment protocol, but the patient also has his or her own assignment and responsibilities as well. Sometimes this combination of efforts and intentions leads to interesting outcomes that would not have emerged otherwise. In both our psoriasis study and in the well-documented outcomes of MBSR, the clinical benefits are in all likelihood dependent on what we might call *presencing*, arising out of embodied moment-by-moment awareness, catalyzed through the cultivation of mindfulness.

The psoriasis study is an example of what eventually came to be called *integrative medicine*, integrative because it integrates mind/body interventions such as meditation right into the delivery of more conventional medical treatments. In this case, the mind/body treatment (the meditation and visualization) is completely co-extensive in time and space with the allopathic treatment (the UV light). You could say that they are orthogonal to each other, occupying the same space at the same time.

It is revealing to note that the subjects in the psoriasis study did not get to take home the guided meditation tapes, nor did they practice in any formal way on their own, unlike in MBSR, where daily practice at home using mindfulness meditation practice tapes or CDs or now digital devices is a required and integral part of the program. This suggests that even very short periods of time practicing meditation, under the right conditions, might have major effects on the body, and presumably on the mind as well. This possibility of even brief periods of engagement in mindfulness practice having a major impact on the mind and body has recently been explored in a number of different studies, with very interesting results.†

---

* See Kabat-Zinn, J. Participatory Medicine. *Journal of the European Academy of Dermatology and Venereology* 14 (2000) 239–240.
† See for example: Zeidan, F. et al. "Mindfulness Meditation Improves Cognition: Evidence of Brief Mental Training." *Consciousness and Cognition* 19 (2010): 597–605.

Parenthetically, MBSR itself could be said to be another example of integrative medicine. First, the Stress Reduction Clinic is an integral part of the Department of Medicine. Doctors from many different departments and subspecialties as well as from internal medicine and primary care refer their patients to it when appropriate as an essential element of their overall treatment plan. Second, it is offered as a well-dovetailed complement to whatever other medical treatments people are already undergoing. One might say that integrative medicine is a harbinger of what good medicine will be in the future. For many medical centers and their patients, that future is, to some degree, already here.

Our study on healing and the mind in people with psoriasis has a number of implications. The most obvious is that the mind can positively influence healing under at least some circumstances. Something that the psoriasis patients in the meditation group were doing or thinking or hoping or practicing was in all likelihood responsible for the faster pace of their skin clearing. It might have been the meditation practice itself, or the visualization, or their expectations or beliefs or intentions, or a combination of all of the above; we won't know for certain until further studies are conducted. But whatever was underlying the accelerated skin clearing we observed, we can say that it was in some way or other related to the activity of the mind.

Another implication is that participatory medicine might be a big money saver in some instances. Our study had the built-in feature of being a de facto cost-effectiveness study. Faster healing means fewer treatments necessary to reach skin clearing, and thus, lower medical charges for the meditators. Since medicine and health care are suffering from ever-escalating costs that even the introduction of HMOs (health maintenance organizations) was only able to stem for a time, the potential to make it easier for medical patients, wherever possible and whenever appropriate, to participate intimately in their own movement toward greater levels of health and well-being as a complement to what the health care system (still at this point in time really primarily a disease care system) might be doing for them, could result in significant and sustained reductions in health care costs, as well as far greater patient satisfaction with their health care, and significant increases in overall mental and physical health and well-being in our society across the lifespan.

What is more, since ultraviolet light is itself a risk factor for skin cancer, fewer treatments would mean less UV exposure, which would mean lowered risk of skin cancer as a side effect of the phototherapy treatments.

And since psoriasis is an example of an uncontrolled cell proliferation, akin in some ways to cancer—in fact, certain genes that are implicated in psoriasis also seem to play a role in basal cell carcinoma—the demonstration that the mind can positively influence skin clearing in the former raises the possibility that the much more dangerous uncontrolled cell proliferation in skin cancer might respond favorably, at least to some degree, to similar meditation practices and motivations.

And finally, since the meditators were alone in the lightbox during their treatments, and were only listening to an audiotape of guided instructions and never even met the person whose voice guided the practices, the results of our study are not likely to be attributable to social support, the well-known and very powerful influence on health and well-being that comes from a sense of belonging to a larger group of people, whether it is family, a church group, an ethnic or cultural group, or even belonging to a temporary community such as a class of patients taking an MBSR program. Because of the phototherapy treatment setup and the isolation of the patients from each other and from even the nurses and doctors while they are in the lightbox, the results are most likely due to the interior mental efforts and attitude of each individual person. For how much social support can there be when you are standing naked and all alone enclosed in a cylindrical lightbox under blistering conditions, with dark goggles on and a pillowcase over your head?

*

Years later, related study compared, not mindfulness practiced individually, as in the psoriasis study, but the group-based MBSR program in its entirety to an active control intervention, that matched MBSR on every one of its features except for the mindfulness training itself. This study looked at what is called neurogenic inflammation. Here, rather than studying people with a chronic inflammatory skin condition such as psoriasis, the researchers induced a painless inflammatory reaction in the laboratory by injecting capsaicin, the component of chili peppers that makes them hot, under the skin of the study participants. Then, after the skin developed a superficial (but not painful) blister in response, the blister size was measured in a systematic way, and the fluid in the inflamed area tested for compounds that promote inflammation, called pro-inflammatory cytokines. This study, conducted by Melissa Rosenkranz, a scientist at the University of Wisconsin's Center for Healthy Minds, who at the time was in Richard Davidson's lab, found that the people in the MBSR program showed a greater decrease in pro-inflammatory cytokines than those in the control group.* She also found, in a related study of long-term mindfulness practitioners, with around 9,000 hours of lifetime practice—remember that in the psoriasis study, the participants were only in the lightbox for minutes at time, three times a week for several weeks, and so had at most one or two hours of total practice time over the course of that study—that experienced meditators also showed smaller patches of inflammation in response to the blister challenge.† Interestingly enough, these subjects were not engaged in a

---

* Rosenkranz, M. A., Davidson, R. J., MacCoon, D. C., Sheridan, J. F., Kalin, N. H., and Lutz, A. A comparison of mindfulness-based stress reduction and an active control in modulation of neurogenic inflammation. *Brain, Behavior, and Immunity* 27 (2013) 174–184.

† Rosenkranz, M. A., Lutz, A., Perlman, D. M., Bachhuber, D.R.W., Schuyler, B. S., MacCoon, D.G., and Davidson, R.J. Reduced stress and inflammatory responsiveness in

meditation program or retreat at the time of this study. This suggests that having a regular ongoing mindfulness practice lessens inflammation day to day, not just while meditating intensively, such as while participating in an MBSR program. In other words, when you cultivate mindfulness in your life on a regular basis, it makes you less prone to inflammatory processes in the body. Since there is strong evidence that inflammation may be an underlying cause of many different chronic diseases, the suggestion is that incorporating mindfulness into everyday living and adopting a regular formal meditation practice might be an effective way to promote greater health across the lifespan, especially in the face of endemic stress. This provides supportive evidence that it is important to take effective measures in your life to counteract the stressful conditions that are often such a large part of our everyday lives.

experienced meditators compared to a matched healthy control group. *Psychoneuoendocrinology* 68 (2016) 117–125.

A Study in Happiness—
Meditation, the Brain, and the
Immune System

We conducted another study in direct collaboration with Richard David-son and his group at of the University of Wisconsin in Madison, to look at the effects of mindfulness on well-being and health. This one looked at some of the effects of MBSR itself, in which, of course, people learn and practice the meditation in fairly large classes, with an instructor, rather than isolated in a lightbox and getting the instructions only from a audiotape, as in the psoriasis study described in the last chapter.

Picture this: Employees at a cutting-edge biotechnology company in Madison were recruited to participate in a study to investigate the effects of meditation on how the brain and immune system respond to stress. All those who volunteered for the study first went through a four-hour period of baseline testing in Davidson's laboratory, where different aspects of brain function were assessed as each individual was challenged by various emotional stimuli while they were engaged in a number of either pleasant or stressful tasks. After this initial test-ing, they were then randomly assigned to be in one of two groups. The first group took the eight-week MBSR program beginning in the early fall of that year. The second group was assigned to wait until the following spring to take the MBSR program. But at the end of the fall, everybody in both groups, those who had completed the pro-gram and those who hadn't yet taken it, were tested again in the lab on the same measures. Then everybody was retested a third time, four months after the second testing.

In this study, the second group served as what is called a wait-list control group, so that we could compare the results of a group of people taking the MBSR program with a group of similar people who hadn't taken it yet.* Although in theory it would have been a good idea to test the effect of the MBSR program on the spring group as well, we did not do that because this was a first attempt at such a study, and it would have been too costly in terms of both time and money.

The company is a progressive one. The CEO, who was instrumental in allowing the study to take place, had agreed to let the program be offered on site during work hours. However, the two and a half hours that people spent in class each week still had to be made up by the participants. This put the fall MBSR group potentially under more stress than those in the wait-list control because they had to juggle their schedules to accommodate the new commitment they had volunteered for.

On top of that, for everybody in both groups there was the stress of going into Dr. Davidson's Laboratory of Affective Neuroscience on those three different occasions for four hours each time. If you were a subject in the study, you would have had to sit in a dark room with a "helmet" of scalp EEG (electroencephalography) electrodes on your head without eating or drinking or going to the bathroom, while technicians put you through a bunch of what can only be described as stressful and emotionally provocative tests to see how your brain would be affected by them. Parts of the testing, like counting backward by threes from one hundred under time pressure while knowing that people are watching your brain activity in that very moment, can be downright humbling.

By way of background, the cerebral cortex, the largest part of our brain and the part that evolved most recently and is involved in all our higher-order cognitive capabilities and emotional processing, has two hemispheres, a left one and a right one. Among countless other functions, the left cerebral hemisphere controls the motor and sensory

---

* The HEP comparison control group which matched MBSR in every respect except the mindfulness was not developed until more than a decade later.

functions on the right side of the body and the right cerebral hemisphere controls those functions on the left side of the body.

Decades of study by Dr. Davidson and his colleagues and by others have shown that a similar brain asymmetry between the left and right hemispheres occurs regarding emotional expression. Activity in specific regions of the frontal and prefrontal cortex (the region of the brain more or less behind the forehead) on the left side tends to be associated with the expression of positive emotions such as happiness, joy, high energy, and alertness. In contrast, activity in similar regions on the right side seems to be activated in the expression of difficult and disturbing emotions, such as fear and sadness. Each of us has a kind of temperamental set point, defined by the baseline ratio between the two sides, which is characteristic of our emotional disposition and temperament. Until this study was conducted, that set point was thought to be pretty much fixed for life.

Interestingly, right-sided activation in these frontal regions of the cerebral cortex is also generally associated with *avoidance*. This is not just true for human beings, but in primates in general and perhaps other mammalian species such as rodents, as well. On the other hand, left-sided activation is associated with *approach*, with pleasure-directed responses. Approach and avoidance . . . two of the most basic behaviors of all living systems, even plants, which don't even have a nervous system. These two characteristics are among our most deeply defining features, since they are so basic to all of life, and since they are also strongly conditioned through experience and social norms. Therefore, we can easily get caught and even hijacked by our habitual and unconscious emotional reactions to various events in our lives, depending on how we interpret the things that happen to us. If an event or situation is perceived as threatening, noxious, or aversive, we tend to avoid it instinctively because our primary motivation is to survive, and our conditioning adds to that instinct. On the other hand, if an event or situation is perceived as pleasurable or nurturing, we will tend to gravitate to it, whether it is something nice to eat, or a feel-good social situation, or just conditions that promise us a bit of peace of mind, because pleasurable experiences give rise to the yearning for more pleasurable experiences, and also to recognizing what might afford us some degree of pleasure. To show that we might be able to exercise a degree of wise control and conscious modulation over these deeply engrained and highly conditioned emotional responses would suggest that mindfulness could be helpful to people in dealing more effectively with some very basic emotional and motivational conditioning related to clinging and aversion that colors virtually everything we do.

For all these reasons, we were particularly interested in seeing what would happen to that temperamental set point in the brain, that ratio of left to right activation in specific regions of the frontal and prefrontal cortex after eight weeks of training in MBSR, especially in a stressful work environment. Would people learn how to handle stress better? Would such changes be reflected in their brains? Could we correlate such changes with biologically significant indicators of health, such as the responsivity of the immune system to exposure to a virus? These were questions we set out to answer in this study. But before coming to what we found, let's consider for a moment some of the challenges involved in doing studies of this kind in the first place.

We were more than a little worried from the outset of our planning process to be doing such an elaborate and expensive study with working people who were basically healthy and who were employed in what can only be described as a gorgeous physical work environment. The clinical effects of MBSR had been established in a hospital setting, with medical patients suffering with chronic illnesses and with stress and pain conditions of all kinds. These patients were referred by their doctors specifically because of these medical conditions, so they were potentially much more highly motivated to throw themselves fully into the practice of meditation and the cultivation of mindfulness than a group of employees who were merely volunteering to participate in a research study. The motivation of these employees stemmed in part from a desire to contribute to expanding our scientific understanding of the brain and emotions, as well as from anticipating some degree of personal benefit from learning new methods for dealing with stress. But I was concerned that these motivations might not be of the same magnitude as the motivation our patients were bringing to their participation in the Stress Reduction Clinic, based on the high levels of emotional and physical distress stemming from outright disease coupled with pervasive dis-ease, in other words, from their ongoing struggles with chronic stress, pain, and illness. Would the company employees be sufficiently motivated to actually practice, rather than just going through the motions?

In fact, on our first visit to the company, when we were given the VIP tour, we had serious concerns about whether the employees, the scientists, technicians, managers, and staff who might participate as subjects in the study, would have any stress to speak of at all, given how stress-free things appeared to be. Here we were, about to embark on a costly study, and with no real pilot data to suggest that there would be any kind of positive response to the MBSR program in this environment, either in terms of the volunteers' motivation to stay in the study and to practice the meditation in a serious way, or in terms of the degree of benefit they might experience, given their apparently low stress levels. Their work environment almost seemed too good to be true, and that might not work to our advantage in conducting a study of this kind.

At the same time, we were also very much aware that human beings are human beings, work is work, and the human mind is the human mind, so we suspected that there might be a good deal more stress in this environment than met the eye. And that, indeed, turned out to be the case.

To return now to the study itself, it wound up showing some interesting things.* Before the meditation training, the groups were indis-

---

* Davidson, R. J., Kabat-Zinn, J., Schumacher, J., Roserkranz, M. S., Muller, D., Santorelli, S. F., Urbanowski, F., Harrington, A., Bonus, K., and Sheridan, J. F. "Alterations

tinguishable in terms of their patterns of brain activation. After eight weeks of training in MBSR, the meditators as a group showed a significant shift to a higher ratio of left- compared to right-sided activation in certain regions, while the control group actually shifted in the opposite direction, to greater right-sided activation.* The higher degree of activation in the left frontal regions of the cerebral cortex in the MBSR group compared to the control subjects was seen both a resting baseline condition and in response to various stressful tasks. These brain changes are consistent with a shift toward more positive emotion and more effective processing of difficult emotions while under stress.

We also found that the shift in the ratio between left and right activation we observed in the meditators at the end of the eight weeks of MBSR training persisted for four months after the training period ended, while no such change was observed in the control group. This suggests that what was thought to be a fixed temperamental set point in the brain controlling the regulation of emotion isn't perhaps so fixed, and can be modulated through the cultivation of mindfulness.

These brain findings at the end of the program and at four-month follow-up were in line with firsthand reports from the meditators of lower trait anxiety (defined as an enduring predisposition toward anxiety) and fewer mental and physical symptoms of stress at both sampling times, compared to when they started.

We also gave everybody in both groups a flu vaccine at the end of the program to see how their immune systems would respond. Would the meditators show a stronger immune response in the form of antibodies produced against the influenza virus in the vaccine than the

---

in brain and immune function produced by mindfulness meditation." *Psychosomatic Medicine* 65 (2003): 564–570.

* Although we cannot know for sure, we interpret this shift of the ratio in the control group in the other direction as perhaps being the result of increasing frustration in these individuals with having to go back into the laboratory for the second and third times to be stressed while people were looking into their brains. Such frustration would be registered as greater right-sided activation compared to left-sided.

control group? In fact, they did. Not only that. When we plotted the degree of change in the brain (the right-to-left shift) versus the antibody response of the immune system in the meditators, we found that there was a linear relationship between the two. The greater the brain change, the greater the immune response. There was no such relationship in the control group.

What does all this mean? It suggests that going through the MBSR program and training in mindfulness and its applications in daily living has measurable consequences that may be important for both mental and physical health. It also shows that people can engage in such a program while at work, under fairly stressful conditions, and still benefit from it, at least in the short term.

It also suggests that meditation training can modulate at least some circuitry responsible for emotional processing in the brain, and is thus an example of the brain's profound neuroplasticity in response to lived experience and training. Since the time of our study, Richie and his colleagues at the Center for Healthy Minds have done an enormous amount of work studying meditators, including monastics with tens of thousands of hours of lifetime meditation practice. These studies and their dramatic findings are described in the book *Altered Traits* by Daniel Goleman and Richard Davidson. As you will find in that book (page 186) the jury is still out on the meaning of the right-to-left shift we observed with MBSR training in our study, since it was never seen in long-term meditators. Our current thinking is that it may be a real finding in beginning meditators because it has been seen since in a number of other studies, and the brain shift in all cases is in the same direction: from right hemisphere to left hemisphere activation. We think it may represent some degree of approach motivation and enthusiasm associated with early stages of regular meditation practice, but which disappears in established meditators. A much more recent study from the same group found that MBSR training can positively affect emotion regulation circuitry in the brain via reduced amygdala reactivity (to positive emotional stimuli) and heightened functional connectivity between the amygdala and a region of the frontal cortex associated with emotion regulation (the ventro-medial prefrontal cortex).*

*

Our study provided early evidence that mindfulness practice could lead to being less caught up in and at the mercy of destructive emotions, and that it predisposes us to greater emotional intelligence and balance, and ultimately, to greater happiness, in addition to the immune system benefits we observed. This happiness, sometimes spoken of as *eudaemonia*, to use Aristotle's word, may be so deep, so much a part of our nature, that it is like the sun, always shining. However, even our strong innate capacity for happiness can be obscured by the cloudiness and the storminess, the weather patterns, so often highly conditioned, of our own minds. Yet, just as the sun is not affected by the weather on Earth, so our innate happiness may remain unaffected by causes and conditions swirling around us in our lives, even if we don't always remember that this is so. Our intrinsic happiness may not always be in evidence in the face of the full catastrophe, but, as our study seemed to show, it may be accessible to some degree at all times, and can be touched, tapped, and brought more into our daily lives through training in mindfulness.

---

* Kral, T.R.A., Schuyler, B. S., Mumford, J. A., Rosenkranz, M. A., Lutz, A., and Davidson, R. J. Impact of short-and long-term mindfulness meditation training on amygdala reactivity to emotional stimuli. *Neuroimage* 181 (2018) 301–313.

Homunculus

We came across this strange word (Latin for "little man," or we could say "little person") before, in Francis Crick's assertion that there is no such entity inside your head that is responsible for and explains the fact of your consciousness—although it can very much feel that way when we get caught up in the sense of I, me, and mine and don't pay too close attention to who we are talking about, or who is thinking such thoughts, or any thoughts at all for that matter.

There is certainly no "little person" of any kind in your head who is perceiving your perceptions, feeling your feelings, and directing your life. There is the inescapable fact and experience of awareness, of sentience, but that, as we have seen, is a huge mystery, and is fundamentally impersonal, unless we choose to cling to the conventional sense of ourselves as an isolated, independent entity, even though, upon examination, it proves to be more illusory than actual.

But interestingly enough, that very same word, "homunculus," plays an important role in neuroscience in spite of what was just said. It is used to describe the various maps of the body in the brain, as you can see in these two drawings.

We touched on this subject in passing when we were visiting the body scan (see Book 2, *Falling Awake*). Your brain has within it a number of what we might call topological maps covering the whole of your body. They are maps in the sense that pretty much every region of the body's surface and its underlying musculature has a corresponding region in the

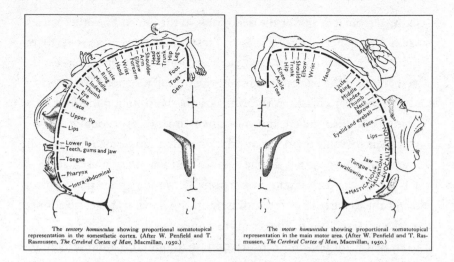

The *sensory homunculus* showing proportional somatotopical representation in the somesthetic cortex. (After W. Penfield and T. Rasmussen, *The Cerebral Cortex of Man*, Macmillan, 1950.)

The *motor homunculus* showing proportional somatotopical representation in the main motor area. (After W. Penfield and T. Rasmussen, *The Cerebral Cortex of Man*, Macmillan, 1950.)

brain that it is connected to and with which it is in intimate and reciprocal relationship. This fact is interesting just to think about, and even more interesting to explore experientially. It's as if the map of the town you live in has direct connections from every location on the map to every single feature in the town itself. Quite an unusual map. What is more, if you didn't have the map, you wouldn't have the town. The possibilities of virtual reality technology will add a whole new dimension to the interplay of maps and experience through simulating any territory imaginable. You could say that evolution figured this out millions of years ago and is continuing to refine it on multiple levels, including our technologies. But perhaps most valuable for our lives and health is the potential to do so through the cultivation of greater awareness of our awareness—of our body, and of everything else in our experiential universe.

One topological map in the cerebral cortex covers the sense of touch. Another covers all areas of the body that are involved in voluntary movement. The sense of touch is located in an area of the brain known as the *somatosensory cortex*, spanning a band that goes across the cerebral cortex from one side of the brain to the other. Voluntary movement lies in what is called the *motor cortex*, at the back of the frontal region, or lobe, in a band right in front of the somatosensory cortex and separated from it by one of the deep folds in the brain. The other senses, such as seeing, hearing, smelling, and tasting, all have other specialized regions of the brain that are primarily responsible for these senses: the visual cortex at the back of the brain (the occipital region), for instance, and the auditory cortex on the sides of the brain (temporal lobes) for hearing. But since touch and movement involve every region of the body, their maps in the brain are the ones that are termed homunculi, because, mapping as they do the surface and voluntary musculature of the body, if you draw them proportionally to the regions they control, you get the distorted figures as drawn on the previous page, positioned over the surface areas of the brain they are related to.

Actually, for both the sensory homunculus and the motor homunculus, there are two maps of each kind, one in each of the two cerebral hemispheres. Recall from the description of the cerebral cortex in the preceding chapter, when we discussed our study of the effects of mindfulness training on the brain and immune system and on the processing of emotion under stress, that there are two major parts to the cerebral cortex, the left hemisphere and the right hemisphere, which are specialized in some ways for different functions.

In the topological maps for either touch sensation or movement, the map in the left hemisphere relates to (or we could say controls) the right side of the body, and the map in the right hemisphere relates to or controls the left side of the body.

The somatosensory and motor cortices were first mapped by the Canadian neurosurgeon Wilder Penfield, in Montreal in the 1940s and 1950s. It was Penfield who discovered that it was possible to draw proportional representations of the body based on the size of each area of the brain devoted to each region of the body. In this way, you actually do get the picture of a little man (or woman), albeit highly distorted because of the different density of motor or sensory neurons innervating various body regions.

Amazingly, Penfield discovered these maps of the body in the brain in the course of performing open brain surgery on over twelve hundred conscious (i.e., not anesthetized) patients with intractable epilepsy who were subject to seizures that could not be controlled with medication. With his patients' permission, Penfield used an electrode to stimulate various regions of the exposed cortex (the exposed brain feels no pain, as there are no sensory nerve endings on the surface of the brain), in part to insure that the surgery he would be doing would not compromise the patients' verbal abilities. In this way, he discovered that stimulation in certain regions produced sensations such as tingling in different parts of the body. By carefully moving the electrode around and getting verbal reports from his conscious patients, Penfield was able to map the entire body onto the surface of the somatosensory cortex, giving rise to the picture of the sensory homunculus.

In other regions, just forward of those that generated these sensations, Penfield found that his electrical stimulation of the brain led to twitching or other movements of muscles in various parts of the body. In this way, gradually mapping the body onto the surface of the motor cortex, the motor homunculus was revealed.

You can see right away from the drawings on page 73 that the map of the body in the brain is not completely contiguous but is broken up in a non-anatomical way. For example, the representation of the hand comes between the face and the head. The genitals map somewhere below the toes. Nor are the maps scaled like the human body. Each looks more like a caricature. The mouth, tongue, and fingers are oversized, while the trunk, arms, and legs are tiny. This is because the map in the brain is related to the number of sensory or motor neurons that are wired in to each region of the body. For instance, we have much more sensation and capacity for discriminating between different kinds of sensations in our hands and fingers, and in our tongue and in our lips (remember that as babies, putting things in our mouths was one of the first ways we got to know the world and our connections with it, the how and the what of what things are) than we do in our arms or legs. And of course, from the point of view of movement, the fingers and hands and the lips and tongue have far greater degrees of freedom in moving, and in subtlety of movement, than do other regions such as the mid back, or the backs of the legs. For the tongue and the mouth, for instance, we might marvel at how readily it can differentiate production of the *c* in Cape from the *c* in Cod, as in Cape Cod. Slightly different. The tongue does it effortlessly, without thinking. Speech and vocalization take a lot of motor innervation.

The size of the various regions of the somatosensory map is also related to the relative importance of the input from that part of the body, and how often it is used. From a survival standpoint, obtaining information from your index finger is more useful than whatever information you might receive from, say, your elbow. By the same token, tactile sensations from the mouth, lips, and tongue are hugely important in the production of intelligible speech, and so occupy more of the map than the back of the head, for instance. This of course enhances the pleasure and sense of connectedness in kissing.

The somatosensory maps of the body in the brain and other maps located in another specialized area of the cerebral cortex, called the *insula*, suggest that whenever we feel a sensation—say, an itch, or a pinprick, or a tingling—somewhere in the body, there is corresponding activity going on in the regions of the somatosensory cortex and the insular cortex that subtend that specific part of the body. We "feel" and "know" where our body is being touched, without even looking, because it is lighting up on our maps of the body in the brain. Without the intimate connections to these representational maps in the cortex, as well as with other regions of the brain that interpret and round out the experience for us and accord it to one degree or another an emotional tone, the bare sensory input from that region by itself will not lead to anything resembling what we experience as feeling, sensing, or knowing. These networks of neurons within the body and the brain contribute the pathways by which we know what and how we feel and where we feel it in the body in any given moment.

Even if you are missing a part of your body, you can still feel it as if it were there because it *is* still there in the map in the brain. If

spontaneous activity in the nerve endings in the stump of an amputated arm or leg stimulates the region of the map to which those nerve
endings are connected, it will generate an experience of the limb
being there, the phantom limb phenomenon.

Recent research has shown that the maps of the body in the brain
are extremely malleable. They reorganize themselves in response to
experiential training, learning, and in the recovery from injury. This is
now referred to as the *plasticity* of the nervous system, or *neuroplasticity*.
In the case of a missing limb or finger, the brain region associated with
that body part can eventually be redeployed to connect with another
adjacent region of the body. The somatosensory cortex actually rearranges itself to accommodate the changed condition of the body. After
a while, stimulating the face or another area near a missing arm might
also stimulate the region of the brain that once subtended the arm and
trigger the experience of the "phantom" limb by this other route.

While having more somatosensory cortex devoted to a body
part might be problematic for someone who is missing a limb, it may
be of potential benefit under other circumstances. It turns out that
brain imaging studies of string musicians show that the region of the
somatosensory cortex that subtends the fingers of the hand that does
the fingering is greatly enlarged compared to the area of their brains
that relate to the hand, that does the bowing. The bowing hand, while
essential to playing, does not experience the same degree of sensory
stimulation to the fingers as does the fingering hand. The same is true
for the index finger that does the reading in Braille readers compared
with the index finger of their other hand.

The general conclusion from a host of extremely interesting
experiments along these lines suggests that cortical maps in humans
and in animals are dynamic, and have the capacity to adjust over time
to changes in experience, especially when they involve repeated use
and learning. This is true not only for the somatosensory cortex but for
the motor cortex and for the visual and auditory cortical maps as well.

In fact, increasing evidence is suggesting that our maps of the body in the brain are extraordinarily dynamic, capable of continually changing over the course of our lives, particularly in response to the activities we engage in on a regular basis over days, weeks, months, and years.*

Not only that. Each map in the brain is highly coordinated and integrated with other brain systems so we can execute refined and complex movements, which require a whole array of different sensory and proprioceptive inputs from moment to moment, such as reaching for and taking hold of an object, or hitting a baseball coming in at close to one hundred miles an hour; or activities requiring fine-motor sensitivity, such as picking up a paper clip; or for moving in ways that embody and convey emotion, such as dancing.

Novel functional brain imaging studies of Buddhist monks and other meditators who have logged tens of thousands of hours of intensive meditation practice, such as the studies mentioned in the last chapter that Richie Davidson and his team at the Center for Investigating Healthy Minds at the University of Wisconsin have been conducting over the past decade and more, are revealing levels of brain activation, coherence, and synchrony across different brain regions, as well as stability of patterns of activation associated with

---

* One example of experience-driven neuroplasticity was shown in a study comparing the brains of experienced London cabdrivers with those in training for the licensing exam required to become a taxi driver in London. The posterior hippocampus in the experienced, licensed drivers was much larger and their anterior hippocampus correspondingly smaller than was the case for those in training to become cabdrivers, who had not yet learned to get around facilely in the medieval maze of London streets. It turns out that the posterior hippocampus plays a major role in spatial orientation. It seems as if it got physically bigger to "contain" the street map of London, and the related knowledge of all the roundabouts, one-way streets, and intricate traffic patterns. Just for fun, imagine if doing the body scan over and over again were to grow and reshape your somatosensory cortex and other associated regions of the brain in a similar way. With years of practice, we of course become intimately more in touch with the body, and the brain may very well be rearranging itself in response to such a daily discipline. Let's not forget that your body is far more complex than the layout of London's streets, that endearingly, the cabdrivers call "the knowledge."

particular meditation practices that were unknown to science even a few years ago.*

Moreover, we have seen already that right-sided brain *activity* in certain regions of the frontal cortex associated with expression of negative or destructive emotions under stress attenuated in people who learned to meditate at work by taking an MBSR course for eight weeks, and that the new pattern endured for up to four months. As we have seen, this finding also points to a possible relationship between meditation practice and neuroplasticity, and of how such brain changes might be mobilized and consolidated over time to beneficial effect through systematic and rigorous training of the mind.

Coming back to the bare experience of sensation, we need to remind ourselves once again that, just as with the other senses, how we actually go from the activation of the nerve endings, say, in the shoulder, that pick up on the sensory stimulus, whatever it is, to the feeling of the sensations *as touch* in that particular region of the body is still a mystery. Cognitive science does not have a full explanation for how the entire body sense is generated, and within it, the individual sensations of various regions. It is part of the mystery of sentience, of how we know what we know, and how we generate an interior experience of a body and the outward experience of an inhabitable world.†

When we practice the body scan, we are systematically and intentionally moving our attention through the body, attending to the various sensations in the different regions. That we can attend to these body sensations at all is quite remarkable, miraculous really, and truly a major mystery when all is said and done. That we can do it at will, either impulsively or in a more disciplined and systematic way, is even

---

* See Goleman, D. and Davidson, R. J. *Altered Traits: Science Reveals How Meditation Changes Your Mind, Brain, and Body* Penguin Random House, New York, 2017.
† See Chomsky, N. *What Kind of Creatures Are We?* Columbia University Press, New York, 2016 (Especially Chapter 2: "What Can We Understand?")

more mysterious. Without moving a muscle, we can put our mind anywhere in the body we choose, and thus feel and be aware of whatever sensations are present in that moment.

Experientially, we might describe what we are doing during a body scan as *tuning in* or *opening* to those sensations, allowing ourselves to become aware of what is already unfolding, much of which we usually tune out because it is so obvious, so mundane, so familiar that we hardly know it is there—I mean here. And of course, by the same token we could say that most of the time in our lives we hardly know we are there—I mean here—*experiencing* the body, *in* the body, *of* the body...the words actually fail the essence of the experience completely. When we speak about it, as we've already observed, language itself forces us to speak of a separate I who "has" a body. We wind up sounding hopelessly dualistic.

And yet, in a way there certainly is a separate I who "has" a body, or at least, there is a very strong appearance and experience of that being the case. We have spoken of this as being characteristic of what we could call *conventional reality*, the relative, the level of appearances. In the domain of relative reality, there is the body and its sensations (object), and there is the perceiver of the sensations (subject). These appear separate and different. They *feel* separate and different.

Then there are moments, and we all have them on occasion, of pure *perceiving*. They arise sometimes in meditation practice, and sometimes at other very special moments in life. Yet such moments are potentially available to us at all times, since they are attributes of awareness itself. Perceiving unifies the apparent subject and the apparent object in the experiencing itself. Subject and object dissolve into awareness. Awareness is larger than sensation. It has a life of its own, separate from the life of the body, yet intimately dependent on it.

As a rule, awareness is deeply bereft, however, when it does not have a full body to work with due to disease or injury, particularly injury to the nervous system itself. The intact nervous system provides us with all of our extraordinary gateways into the feeling, sensing world. Yet, like most everything else, we take these capacities so much for granted that we hardly notice that every exquisite moment of our life unfolding in relationship to experience, both inwardly and outwardly, depends on them. Not only might we benefit from literally coming to our senses a great deal more than we usually do. We might realize that we only know through our senses, if you include the mind, or awareness itself, as a sense—you could say, the ultimate sense.

When we are scanning the body region by region in the body scan meditation, it should by now be obvious that we are *de facto* simultaneously and intimately scanning the map of the body in the somatosensory cortex and in other areas of the brain, such as the insula. The maps and the "body" are not separate from each other. They are not actually different "things" but part of one seamless whole that we experience (words fail here once again) as the body when we are actually in touch with it. We might have no experience of sensation, or very different experiences of sensation, if either the maps or the body itself were damaged, or the connections between them severed.

Yet the introduction of awareness into the mix somehow enhances sensation, and also the integration of the brain and body and a larger perspective on experience itself. At least it feels that way. Perhaps the somatosensory cortex really is rearranging itself in response to regular meditation practice of this sort. We certainly *experience* our awareness of the body growing more refined, more subtle, more sensitive, more vivid and stable, more nuanced emotionally as we tune to the various dimensions of the bodyscape. And that feeling is supported anecdotally by the large numbers of medical patients training in mindfulness who report profound changes in their *relationship* to chronic pain conditions, or to cancer or heart disease, to their experience of fear, and to their view of their bodies from doing the body scan every day over a period of several weeks.

It is not uncommon while practicing the body scan for the sensations in the body to be felt more acutely, even for there to be more pain, a greater intensity of sensation in certain regions. At the same time, in the context of mindfulness practice, the sensations, whatever they are and however intense, are also being *met* more acutely and more accurately too, with less overlay of interpretation, judgment, and reaction, including aversion and the impulse to run, to escape.

In the body scan, we are developing a greater intimacy with bare sensation, opening to the give-and-take embedded in the reciprocity between the sensations themselves and our awareness of them. As a result, it is not uncommon to be less disturbed by them, or disturbed by them in a different, perhaps wiser way, even when they are acute. Awareness learns to let sensations in the body be as they are and to hold them without triggering so much emotional reactivity, and also so much inflamed thinking about them. We sometimes speak of awareness and discernment *differentiating* and perhaps naturally *"uncoupling"* the sensory dimension of the experience of pain from the emotional and cognitive dimensions of pain. In the process, the intensity of the sensations themselves can sometimes subside. In any event, these sensations may come to be experienced as less onerous, less debilitating, and sometimes even, less defining and confining of one's life.

It seems as if awareness itself, embracing and holding the sensations without judging them or reacting to them, can heal our view of the body and allow it to come to terms, at least to some degree, with conditions as they are in the present moment in ways that no longer overwhelmingly erode our quality of life, even in the face of pain or disease. The awareness of the experience of "intense discomfort" is really a different realm entirely from being caught up in the pain and struggling with it. Setting foot in that realm to whatever degree we might be able to in any given moment, even tentatively at first, we discover some succor and respite. This in itself is an experience of liberation, a profound freedom in that moment at least from a narrower way of holding the experience of pain when it is not seen as bare sensation. It is not a cure by any means, but it is a learning and an opening, an accepting of sensory experience as it is in that moment, and a navigating of the ups and downs of what previously was impenetrable and unworkable.

What we say to the people coming to MBSR, whatever their situation, whatever the condition that they find themselves in, whatever the pain and the suffering they have been carrying, however much despair they may be in, is that, in giving themselves over wholeheartedly to the meditation practices, they will very likely come to see that their situation is at least somewhat workable. And sometimes, that "somewhat" is huge, and hugely revealing.

Life responds to our cultivation of wise attention in remarkable ways, perhaps in part because of the deep plasticity of the nervous system. But wise attention requires that, when faced with great life challenges, especially those that bring with them enormous suffering and grief, we be willing, in the face of all our pain and turmoil and even feelings of despair, to do a certain kind of work on and with ourselves, a work that no one on the planet can do for us, no matter how much they might want to, no matter how much love they have for us, no matter how badly they feel for us, no matter how much they are helping us in the ways that they can be of help.

Things in the domain of inner and outer experience are workable to an astonishing degree, but much more so and sometimes *only* if you step up and do the work. It may be the most difficult work in the world, and I for one believe that, when it comes to cultivating mindfulness and tasting freedom from the conditioned mind, it actually is the most difficult work in the world.

But in the end, what else is there to do? It is your very life that hangs in the balance, and for that reason alone, the work is profoundly satisfying in addition to being so challenging. We discover that it is indeed intrinsically fulfilling to be fully present, to attend non-reactively, nonjudgmentally, even, or, especially, when what we might be attending to is fear, or loneliness, or confusion and the psychic pain that accompanies such mind states. We discover that such mind states and body states are indeed workable, and that means, ultimately, profoundly healable.

When I am practicing the body scan, whether I am experiencing pain in the body at the time or not, I sometimes get the feeling that in scanning the body—and thus, as we have seen, the somatosensory cortex and other related maps that generate the feeling of being "in" the body—I am actually *feeding* my brain, exercising it in a way that is similar to my dog's exercising her olfactory cortex when she sniffs the world. So, in my own life, I stick with the body scan and awareness of my breathing at times, and to giving myself over to all my senses, however acute or paltry. Meanwhile, she sniffs her way around in the fields and along the roads. My highways and byways are the pathways of proprioception and interoception, the felt sense of the body's presence and position in space and its internal condition, and, of course, what the mind is up to in any moment. I can rejoice in putting my awareness in my feet, in my ankles, in my knees, my legs, my pelvis, the whole of the body as it lies here. It feeds me and, no doubt, it tunes the somatosensory cortex, maybe even excites it, or activates it, as the neurobiologists might say. Maybe certain regions of the somatosensory cortex and related areas are even growing in size from these regular visitations.

Whether future studies show that to be the case or not, I would say it's a good thing to develop those connections, to befriend the homunculi, to massage the sensory cortex and the motor cortex, and feed the nervous system. I would say it's a good thing to train the mind to inhabit the body, to let our experience of being alive be co-extensive with the body, enfolded into body, not as a fixed state but as a vital and dynamic moment-to-moment flow.

In this way, the experience of being embodied has a chance to develop into a robust, reliable feeling, no longer perpetually at risk of being eviscerated by the dullness of our habitual ignoring or discounting of what is familiar and closest to home, which can in the end only cut us off from our own life and possibilities, and imprison us in a profound alienation from nature and from our own interiority.

Paraphrasing James Joyce in one of his short stories in *Dubliners*, "Mr. Duffy lived a short distance from his body." That may be an address too many of us share. Taking the miracle of embodiment for granted or ignoring it altogether is a horrific loss. It would be a profound healing of our lives to get back in touch with it.

All it takes is practice in coming to our senses, all of them.

And...a spirit of adventure.

Proprioception—The Felt Sense of the Body

We know that it is possible to lose the felt sense of the body or parts of it through traumatic injury. In spinal cord injuries, the nerves communicating between the body and the brain can be severely injured or severed completely. In such situations, as a rule, the person is paralyzed as well as being unable to feel his or her body in those areas controlled by the spinal nerves below the break. Both the sensory and the motor pathways between brain and body and body and brain are affected. The actor Christopher Reeve, who died in 2004, sustained such an injury to his neck when he was thrown from a horse. We will take up his remarkable story in the next chapter.

A number of years ago, the neurologist Oliver Sachs, who died in 2015, described meeting a young woman who had lost only the sensory dimension of bodily experience due to an unusual and very rare polyneuritis (inflammation) of the sensory roots of her spinal and cranial nerves. This inflammation, unfortunately, extended throughout the woman's nervous system. It was caused, in all likelihood and quite horrifically, by treatment with an antibiotic administered prophylactically in the hospital in advance of routine surgery for gallstones.

All this woman, whom Sachs called Christina, was left being able to feel was light touch. She could sense the breeze on her skin riding in an open convertible and she could sense temperature and pain, but even these she could only experience to an attenuated degree. She had lost all sense of having a body, of being in her body, of what is technically called *proprioception*, which Sachs calls "that vital sixth sense without which a body must remain unreal, unpossessed." Christina had no muscle or tendon or joint sense whatsoever, and no words to describe her condition. Poignantly, in the same way that we saw for people who lack sight or hearing, she could only use analogies derived from her other senses to describe her experiences.*

"I feel my body is blind and deaf to itself . . . it has no sense of itself." In Sachs's words, "she goes out when she can, she loves open cars, where she can feel the wind on her body and face (superficial sensation, light touch, is only slightly impaired)." "It's wonderful," she says. "I feel the wind on my arms and face, and then I know, faintly, I *have* arms and a face. It's not the real thing, but it's something—it lifts this horrible dead veil for a while."

Along with the loss of her sense of proprioception came the loss of what Sachs calls the fundamental mooring of identity—that embodied sense of being, of having a corporeal identity. "For Christina there is this general feeling—this 'deficiency in the egoistic sentiment of individuality'—which has become less with accommodation with the passage of time." Amazingly, she found her senses of sight and hearing assisting her with reclaiming some degree of external control over the positioning of her body and its ability to vocalize, but all her movements have to be carried out with extreme deliberateness and conscious attention. All the same, "there is this specific, organically based, feeling of disembodiedness, which remains as severe, and uncanny, as the day she first felt it." Unlike those who are paralyzed by transections high up in the spinal cord who also lose proprioception, "Christina, though 'bodiless,' is up and about."

Make no mistake about it. Just as the loss of knowing who you are in sufferers of Alzheimer's disease is in no way some kind of shortcut to selflessness, the loss of this proprioceptive mooring is not liberating

---

* See "The Disembodied Lady," in *The Man Who Mistook His Wife for a Hat*, a compilation of clinical histories from Sachs's neurology practice.

in any sense of the word. It is not enlightenment, nor a dissolving of ego, nor the letting go of an overwrought attachment to the body. It is a pathological, utterly destructive process that robs the individual of what Sachs calls, quoting the philosopher Ludwig Wittgenstein, "the start and basis of all knowledge and certainty." We have no words to describe the feelings we might be left with in the face of such a loss because the loss of the felt sense of the body, especially when the body can still move, is inconceivable to us.

> Those aspects of things that are most important for us are hidden because of their simplicity and familiarity. (One is unable to notice something because it is always before one's eyes.) The real foundations of his enquiry do not strike a man at all.

These are Wittgenstein's words, with which Sachs opens his story about that "sixth sense" we so don't know we have, so much is it in evidence, namely the felt sense of the body in space. It is so allied with our physicality, our physical "presence," our sense of the body as proper to us and therefore as our own, that we fail to notice it or appreciate its centrality in our construction of the world and who we (think we) are.

When we practice the body scan, our awareness includes that very sense of proprioception that Sachs is describing and that Christina tragically lost, the felt sense of having a body and, within the universe of the body as one seamless whole, the felt sense of all its various regions, which we can isolate in our minds to a degree, zero in on, and "inhabit." When we practice the body scan, we are reclaiming the vibrancy of the body as it is from the cloud of unawareness that stems from its being taken for granted, so familiar is it to us. Without trying to change anything, we are investing it with our attention and therefore, with an embodied sense of appreciation and our love. We are explorers of this mysterious, ever-changing body-universe that simultaneously is us in such a profound way and isn't us in an equally profound way.

And when some sort of healing is longed for and remains a possibility, however remote it might seem, a willingness to reclaim the body from the oblivion of taken-for-grantedness or from narcissistic self-obsession is paramount. Working at it every day, we reconnect with the very source of our humanity, with our elemental core of being.

When awareness embraces the senses it enlivens them. We have all felt that at times, moments of extraordinary vividness. In the case of proprioception, when we truly give ourselves over to *listening* to the body in a disciplined and loving way and persevere at it for days, weeks, months, and years as a discipline and as a love affair in and of itself, even if we don't hear much at first, there is no telling what might occur. But one thing is sure. As best it can, the body is listening back, and responding in its own mysterious and profoundly enlivening and illuminating ways.

NEUROPLASTICITY AND THE
UNKNOWN LIMITS OF THE POSSIBLE

The difficult we do today. The impossible takes a little longer.

MOTTO OF THE U.S. ARMY CORPS OF ENGINEERS

I like to think that, rather than reflecting an arrogant, militaristic, macho attitude saturated with hubris, this motto of the army's corps of engineers reflects the potential power of a truly open mind and a can-do attitude, a willingness to tackle situations that our old conditioned habits of mind may label as impossible way too prematurely. Many times, even in our own personal experience, our minds have surely thought something or other to be impossible that was later shown to be possible and that contributed in some way to our well-being or edification.

Let's not forget that crossing the ocean was once thought to be impossible. Flying was once thought to be impossible. Ending apartheid and instituting democracy in South Africa without a terrible race war was once thought to be impossible.

As Emily Dickinson put it:

I dwell in Possibility—
A fairer House than Prose—
More numerous of Windows—

Superior—for Doors—
Of Chambers as the Cedars—
Impregnable of eye—
And for an everlasting Roof
The Gambrels of the Sky—
Of Visitors—the fairest—
For Occupation—This—
The spreading wide my narrow Hands
To gather Paradise—

We never really know what might be possible in the mindscape and the bodyscape, even in the face of a major injury or disease and the huge damage and dis-regulation that can follow in their wake. This is especially true when those seemingly insurmountable challenges we are presented with, whatever they are, are embraced with utter attention and intentionality.

Take the case of the late Christopher Reeve, the actor and director best known professionally for his work portraying Superman. His tenacity, determination, and his generosity of spirit in light of what befell him seem oddly and uniquely appropriate to that appellation (Superman) from which he was unable to escape. Paralyzed from the neck down after a horseback riding accident in 1995, Mr. Reeve had been told repeatedly by his doctors that he would never be able to move any part of his body below the neck. His situation was described as a "worst-case scenario." But, in the words of Dr. Michael Merzenich of UCSF, a pioneer in neuroplasticity research and the changes that can occur in brain maps in the somatosensory cortex and the auditory cortex due to learning and repeated use, Christopher Reeve "called into question every assumption about the capacity of the human brain and spinal cord to recover after catastrophic injury."

The dogma of neurology until very recently was that it was impossible to recover from severe neurological spinal cord damage because the disrupted or severed nerve cells cannot grow back or reconnect to reestablish conduction pathways for nerve impulses between the body and the brain. These pathways have to be intact for the motor cortex and other movement centers in the brain to control the muscles of the body, and for the body to give proprioceptive feedback about what is happening in movement, and to convey touch-related sensation of any kind to the somatosensory cortex and other brain centers responsible for making sense of the physical world. But the experience of Christopher Reeve and of others with spinal cord injuries and stroke damage are now, through the changes they are experiencing as a result of novel forms of therapy, belying this dogma and fomenting a quiet revolution in rehabilitation medicine. They are also extending the clinical implications and relevance of neuroplasticity for the body and its sensory and motor functions.

In Mr. Reeve's case, at least three-quarters of the nerve fibers in his spinal cord at the level of the neck were severed by the injury, and what remained did not work. He was totally paralyzed from the neck down, unable to feel or move anything, or even to breathe without a ventilator because the injury also affected the nerves that control the diaphragm. For the first five years following the accident, he made use of passive electrical stimulation to maintain his muscle mass and increase circulation. He also spent time lying on a table that tilted him vertically to increase bone density and further enhance circulation. And he tried hanging suspended in a harness over a moving treadmill. All these efforts to reawaken his body were of no avail clinically. He saw no improvements. But he refused to give up.

After five years of no change in his physical status and a great many life-threatening medical complications, Mr. Reeve undertook, with the help of his physicians and caregivers, what can only be described as a super-human exercise program, known as "activity-based recovery," or ABR. In this program, his body was passively moved on a recumbent stationary bicycle by computer-assisted electrical stimulation of major muscle groups in his legs. He underwent this training for one hour per day, three days per week at a fixed level of output (three thousand revolutions per hour). In addition, he underwent daily electrical stimulation of major muscle groups in the arms and trunk on a rotating schedule. At a certain point, aquatic therapy was introduced once a week, in which he could move and be moved by a physical therapist in a pool and work dynamically with the resistance of the water without having to struggle as much with gravity. He also began training in breathing exercises. Reeve kept at this intense passively assisted exercise program because, he says, it kept his muscles strong and his mood elevated.

One morning, after almost six years of no sensation in his body and no voluntary control of movement, and almost one year after starting the intensive ABR program, he found that he could voluntarily control a spastic twitching movement in his left index finger.

That tiny beachhead into the possibility of movement was the start of a slow rebirth of both sensation and motor control over the next three years. Reflecting on that day, he said, "My first reaction was to curb my enthusiasm. But inside, my hope and belief was that if my finger could suddenly move on command, I had to explore every other part of my body to see what was possible. . . . That's when I decided to exercise even more intensively."

Keep in mind that in saying this, Mr. Reeve was even more lacking in proprioceptive experience below the neck than Christina in the preceding chapter. So when he speaks of "my body" it was at the time more a thought and a memory than a present-moment relationship . . . that is, until the finger moved.

In moving, a new level of connection arose. It became "his" finger again, rather than a sense-devoid immobile appendage that could be seen but not felt, and that was entirely unresponsive to his will. In moving under his control that day, the finger came back to life, one might say. And in the years that followed, more and more of his body came back to life. Sadly, in the midst of these optimistic developments, he died suddenly of cardiac arrest in 2004, at the age of 52.

Imagine the faith, resolve, discipline, and unrelenting focus of mind necessary to keep exercising a body that one cannot feel, day in, day out for months and months with no discernible "progress" while at the same time, metaphorically speaking, swimming upstream against the prevailing clinical view dictating against there ever being any.

Yet, as the clinical report attests, Reeve's progress during that time was extraordinary. In the years following the start of his activity-based recovery program, he improved by two grades on the scale of spinal cord injury, a degree of improvement never seen before in any person with an injury as severe as his. Early responses included dramatic benefits to his body even in the absence of improved function. These included increased muscle mass and bone density, and cardiovascular endurance, as well as decreased muscle spasticity. These physical changes vastly improved Mr. Reeve's health and quality of life during that time. The incidence of infections requiring antibiotics decreased dramatically. His severe osteoporosis, which contributed to pathological fractures of two of the largest bones in his body, the femur and the humerus, was completely reversed and brought back to the level he was at before his accident.

Somewhat later, he began seeing what the doctors call functional improvements, in other words, recovery of sensation and motor control, starting with the day he could move his finger. These changes continued to build. By twenty-two months into the exercise program, light touch sensation had improved to 52 percent of normal, and within another six months it had gone up to 66 percent of normal. In addition to recovery of light touch and pinprick (pain) sensations, there was recovery of the ability to perceive vibration, an ability to differentiate heat from cold, and amazingly, a recovery of his sense of proprioception, which allowed him to know when his position needed to be changed to avoid skin irritation and breakdown due to cutting off of blood flow. At the time of a clinical report in the medical literature published by his doctors in

2002,* about 70 percent of Reeve's body was actively represented in his brain, which means that sensory information was once again flowing to his cortex from the periphery, in other words, from his skin and muscles and bones and joints, and that motor messages were flowing from his motor cortex to his arms and legs, and to other parts of his body.

There was also a twenty-point improvement (from 0 to 20 on a scale of 0 to 100) in motor scores, which translated into movement in most joints, including the elbows, wrists, fingers, hips, and knees. Most muscles in the legs were not yet able to oppose gravity, but standing and even walking in the pool became possible, and he could work at exercising his arm, leg, and trunk muscles on his own against appropriate levels of resistance. He was also able to breathe without the ventilator for more than an hour at a time, even though he was still dependent on it.

"What I think happened by exercising over a long period of time," Reeve said, "is that dormant pathways have reawakened." His doctors agreed, and attempted to develop theories to explain his progress in response to his intensive exercise program, along the same lines that complex neurological circuitry is known to develop in infants and children in response to movement. This natural plasticity of the nervous system slows way down in adulthood, but apparently it does not turn off altogether. According to his neurologist, Dr. John W. McDonald, of Washington University School of Medicine in St. Louis, Missouri, many spinal cord injuries leave some ascending (toward the brain from the body) and descending (toward the body from the brain) nerve tracts alive but stunned. Without activity, these fibers atrophy and the person ends up in a wheelchair. But when the muscles are stimulated with electrodes and exercise, the nerve tracts sometimes partly revive.

One way to drive plasticity in the adult brain and body is to break down what has to be learned into small steps. The activity also has to matter to the individual, according to Dr. Merzenich. If it is boring

---

* McDonald, J. W., Becker, D., et al., "Late Recovery Following Spinal Cord Injury." *Journal of Neurosurgery: Spine* 97 (2002): 252–265.

and mindless, the brain's plasticity mechanisms will not kick in. When a person focuses and pays attention, brain molecules turn on the reward circuitry that promotes plasticity, according to a report in the *New York Times* (September 22, 2002).

Before he died, Mr. Reeve's level of recovery had had a life-altering impact on him. In his physicians' report eight years following his accident, three years after beginning the activity-based recovery program, Reeve noted that he was able to stay out of the hospital for more than three and a half years. "Before that, I had blood clots, pneumonia, a collapsed lung, very serious decubitus ulcers (pressure sores), and an infected ankle which threatened amputation of my leg. I was always very tentative about my life because I never knew what would go wrong next. Over the last couple of years, I have become very confident with my health. I have been able to stay off antibiotics. My weight is under control. I can stay up in the chair for as much as fifteen or sixteen hours without a problem. Given the fact that I am a ventilator-dependent C2 [spinal cord injury level], I would say that I am probably in the best possible condition. I am able to work and travel in a way that is very satisfying. The next incremental goal will be to get off the ventilator."

He did, for a while, after undergoing an experimental surgical procedure to install a diaphragm stimulator, essentially a pacemaker for the lungs, which allows him to breathe without the respirator for periods of time and strengthen the muscles of the diaphragm. And as a result, he was able to breathe through his nose and mouth for the first time in eight years and speak normally without the respirator. He also recovered his sense of smell, which had been entirely lost after the accident, and easily identified the fragrances of coffee, mint, and oranges when tested by his medical team.

"I would like more useful functional recovery. I am able to move my arms, fingers, and legs, and yet, I am still sitting in this wheelchair. I hope I will be able to get incremental recovery along those lines so I can be in a different wheelchair, and I could have more freedom, be less dependent on others than I am now."

He went on to say, "My life's goals are more attainable now because I can tell the producer of a film that I can travel to a location to direct, which is my profession. To give speeches, which is part of my profession. I can be counted on. In the past, infection or other illness would prevent me from fulfilling my obligations. It is a great relief to know I can make a commitment and keep it because of my health.

"The impact [of my recovery] on my daily life has been increased mobility and respiratory benefits. A ventilator failure back in 1995, '96, '97 would have been a terrifying experience because I really couldn't breathe. Now, I can breathe quite well. When I breathe, I use the correct technique. I am able to move my diaphragm, an ability that was achieved by exercise and training. That is the most comforting aspect of my recovery, that safety factor.

"Sensation has improved from nothing below the neck to about 65% [of normal]. What is so important about sensation is contact with other people. It makes a huge difference if someone touches you on the hand and you can feel it. You make a much more meaningful connection.

"I look on building muscle mass as preparation for recovery, which is the long-term goal. But more importantly, muscle mass is essential to any movements you need to make, to keep your cardiovascular system working well, and it also relates to maintaining adequate bone density. Let's say you have very weak leg muscles. Standing on a tilt table would be dangerous for the bones in your legs because they don't have enough support. I went through that. I did not know that I had severe osteoporosis. Through exercise and an intense course of calcium, I have completely reversed osteoporosis. I have the bones back that I did when I was thirty. [Reeve was almost fifty at the time of the interview.] It is important that the medical system knows that osteoporosis can be reversed in spinal cord injury. But also, in terms of my self-image, to look down at my legs and not see noodles is very important. In fact, my leg and biceps dimensions are almost the same as before the injury. This is seven years later, so that does a lot to make me feel better about myself.

"I am able to go out with the family... and watch my kids and friends play. I can be as close as I can [get] to the site without participating, but I have also learned how to get satisfaction out of watching my family and friends do leisure activities. So, I am there and a part of it even though I can't do it the way that I used to.

"I feel that the progress made so far is symbolic of the progress that is yet to come... I want to recover to as near normal as possible and I hold that dream. I don't want to let go of it and perhaps a psychological indicator of what I believe is that in the seven years since my injury, I have never had a dream in which I am disabled. I want my life back."

By April of 2004, Reeve had experienced a number of disheartening setbacks. His body rejected the diaphragm pacing unit after a series of infections and pneumonia, and as a result, he had to be put back on the respirator. He could no longer exercise in the pool and was unable to continue his recovery program. He was also unable to exercise on a treadmill, as his femur snapped in half due to osteoporosis the first time he tried it, and he had to have a metal plate and fifteen screws installed in his leg. But he never gave up hope, taking some pleasure in knowing that he was a pioneer whose experience was able to help those requiring similar procedures after spinal cord injuries. He pointed out that he was only the second person in the world to receive a diaphragmatic pacing implant, and while it didn't work for him, what was learned in his case made it possible for the next seven patients to all get off their ventilators. His experience also contributed to making routine the screening of spinal cord injury patients for osteoporosis before allowing them to work out on the treadmill. He took pleasure and comfort in having been able to affect the quality of life of other people in similar situations.

It was quite apparent at the time that Reeve was not pursuing his recovery program only for himself. He became a major spokesperson and inspiration for people with spinal cord injuries, delivering the message that "life doesn't end with physical injury and that they can still live a full and interesting life." In his last years, Reeve established a foundation to further research, and regularly lobbied Congress to support more research into treating spinal cord injuries and paralysis. In spite of his obvious limitations, he persisted in traveling widely to meet with people and families who are affected by spinal cord injuries, and to give public talks.

As with all of us, Christopher Reeve did not know what the limits of the possible were for him. To the end, he remained unwavering in his determination to stay the course and work at the boundaries of the possible for his body and his mind from moment to moment and from day to day, keeping his long-term goals in mind, but focusing on today and the challenges of this moment. Given the level of loss in his life, and the impediments and setbacks he experienced, he could have easily fallen into despair, hopelessness, self-pity, and isolation. That he took on the challenge to work with his situation and to maintain hope and to stay grounded in his love relationships and in his work is moving testimony to the powers of mind and body to heal when they work in concert with the appropriate medical care and support, and with imaginative attempts to mobilize and trust in and amplify the body's natural capacities for self-regulation and repair, even when a positive outcome is uncertain or all but denied as a possibility.

And Mr. Reeve was not alone. People who have suffered spinal cord injuries, strokes, or other neurological damage are making unexpected progress at treatment centers around the world, using novel rehab methods, such as, for example, immobilizing a functional arm so that the patient is forced to use the damaged arm for everyday tasks, or suspending the patient in a harness while his or her feet are put through walking movements on a treadmill. Rehabilitation medicine is even making use of robots to help paralyzed patients practice walking. Using such techniques, thousands of paraplegics who had limited sensations in their lower bodies and no motor function are now able to walk for short distances, unassisted, or using walkers, a remarkable milestone on the path of "learning to live inside again," the deep meaning of the word "rehabilitation."

Is there a take-home message here for those of us who are relatively able-bodied by comparison? I think so. Aerobic and musculoskeletal exercises that keep the body fit and regulated obviously tone and fine-tune the nervous system as much as they do the muscles. There is no doubt that this is true at any age, and is especially important to remember as we age. But beyond exercise, the bringing together of attention, determination, and love of life to work at the very edges of our physical and emotional capacities may be the secret ingredient in seeing our situation as workable, whatever it is, and in putting in the work and the love to allow us to live the lives that are ours to live, never giving up on ourselves and what might be possible if we stay the course and stay in touch through thick and thin, with what is most important. Ultimately, when cultivated deliberately and, as in Reeve's case, through sheer determination and willpower, the willingness to work at the boundary of what is possible in any and every moment and be present to it with patience, determination, humility, and great attention, constitutes the core of mindfulness practice. It exemplifies the motivation required to stay the course for its own sake, and thereby continue growing in one way or another, or in many different ways simultaneously.

Reeve's faith was in relationality and reciprocity—with his body, with his family and his friends, with his professional calling—even when he could not feel the physical touch of others and when his body did not talk back to him. In taking responsibility for and accepting his condition after the accident and working with it as it was, as best he could, with utter perseverance and resolve and a great deal of help over the years, he exemplified perseverance and faith in what might be possible, while not denying the day-in, day-out emotional difficulties and utter disruption associated with his paralysis, which radically changed the lives of all his family members and their relationships.* I heard Reeve say in a public talk in April 2004, six months before he died, "When things aren't going all that well, I still stick to the discipline, no matter what. There is a tremendous ability within our minds to affect the body."

*

I think it is worth noting before we close out this chapter that 2018 saw the death of another intrepid individual who lived far longer than anyone thought he would, and who also showed incredible tenacity and commitment to living as fully as possible in the face of an unimaginably debilitating and potentially demoralizing disease. I am talking about Stephen Hawking, the British theoretical physicist and cosmologist who from his early twenties suffered with amyotrophic lateral sclerosis (Lou Gehrig's Disease) and yet lived to the age of 76 (he was told when he was twenty-one years old that he had only a few years to live), doing his work from a wheelchair that, with the progression of the disease, he ultimately controlled only with his little finger and voluntary eye movements, and using those eye movements coupled with a computerized voice synthesizer to speak. Yet his mind, untouched by the disease, contributed to major breakthroughs and insights into some of the most profound areas of physics and cosmology, most notably the discovery that black holes give off radiation, now known as Hawking radiation, and thus will ultimately explode and return their substance and energy to the surrounding universe. He lived in a body that would be unimaginably

---

* And not denying the day-in, day-out emotional difficulties and rending associated with such a situation. Reeve's wife, Dana, was quoted as saying, "I don't want to be perceived only as this doting, pure saintly wife who would do anything for her man. That is part of me, but I am also many other things. I am in love with and loyal to him and I feel a sense of duty which I knew existed the day I said 'I do.' His physical care is now the responsibility of nurses. I have removed myself from that because we need to be husband and wife, not patient and care-giver." (May 3, 2003, interview in *The Daily Mail*, UK—from the Internet)

challenging for any human being to inhabit—imagine not being able to move any part of your body except a finger and your eyes—yet managed to live a full life, marry, have children, write books, engage improbably in many playful and even risky pursuits* and became a "celebrated pop culture icon," as described by the *New York Times* in his obituary, and often spoken of in the same breath as Albert Einstein. Hawking said, when asked why he engaged in such risky and challenging pursuits: "I want to show people need not be limited by physical handicaps as long as they are not disabled in spirit." He also said: "When you are faced with the possibility of an early death, it makes you realize that life is worth living and that there are a lot of things you want to do." His ashes were buried in Westminster Cathedral, between the remains of Isaac Newton, whose chair he held at Cambridge University, and Charles Darwin.

*

For a brief period of time in the early 2000s, I got to know a young college professor, Philip Simmonds, who had the same disease as Hawking and who, with support from his family and a community of friends and neighbors, managed to find a way to, as he put it so eloquently and poignantly, "learn to fall."† He too found a way to dwell in possibility, right up to the end, at age 44.

*

When Emily Dickinson invoked that wholehearted affirmation of all that is mysterious, transcendent, and sacred, "I dwell in possibility," we saw that she coupled it in the very next line with "A fairer

---

* Such as at age 65, taking part in a zero-gravity-simulating flight on a Boeing 747, and hoping to actually ride a rocket ship into space, something he did not live to accomplish. Hardly any able-bodied people would be able to manage such adventures.

† Simmonds, P. *Learning to Fall: The Blessings of an Imperfect Life*, Bantam, New York, 2003.

house than prose." I take "prose" to mean the domicile of the reasonable, the rational, the linear, those often self-limiting thoughts and opinions we harbor that so convincingly tell us what we can't do, and which, thereby, make the impossible impossible, when it truly isn't.

How about our own minds, and our own sometimes unwanted or terrifying circumstances, and when we find ourselves on occasion face-to-face with the unthinkable when it is already here?

Might we say the same? Might we too find ways to assert that we dwell in possibility? That we too can dwell in the uncertainty of not knowing but still take life-affirming risks in the face of the naysayers in the form of both our own inner discouraging voices and those of others?

How about now, in this very moment? How about with things exactly as they are—giving up for a moment having to have them be any different at all?

How does it feel?

PART 2

Arriving At Your Own Door

*The time will come
When, with elation,
You will greet yourself arriving
at your own door...*

Derek Walcott, from "Love After Love"

"I CAN'T HEAR MYSELF THINK!"

Did you ever hear yourself blurt out something like that? That string of words usually issues forth in frustration when there is a lot of noise in the room and we are trying to concentrate. It means something like "I can't think straight, I can't focus. Will you all please pipe down?!"

But when we sit down to meditate and drop into some degree of stillness, it is amazing... sometimes all there is is hearing yourself think, and it can be louder and more disturbing and distracting than any external noise! The roar of our thinking can be deafening and seemingly endless. It can prevent any kind of stable focus or concentration. It also completely obscures the underlying peace and silence that are to be found right beneath this tumult in the mind once the mind has learned or trained itself to settle down and be still, or stiller.

If we begin to listen to the stream of thought as thought, to attend to thoughts as events in the field of awareness, as we do when we undertake to cultivate mindfulness through formal meditation practice, as described in Book 2 of this series, *Falling Awake,* and if we develop a certain calmness and quiet outwardly, we can actually come to observe our thinking much more clearly. We are able to listen to it, attend to it, recognize each thought as just that, a thought rather than the truth, and thus come to see exactly what is on our minds, and how much of it is just mental noise. Once we know that, intimately, up-close and personal, we can begin to develop new ways of relating to it.

We may be shocked at what we discover, at how much of our

thinking is chaotic and yet at the same time severely narrow and repetitive, shaped so much by our history and habits. Yet it is probably better to know this via firsthand experience than not to know it. When unattended, our thinking runs our lives without our even knowing it. Attended in awareness, we have a chance not only to know ourselves better, and see what is on our minds, but also to hold our thoughts differently, so they no longer rule our lives. In this way, we can taste some very real moments of freedom that do not depend entirely on inner or outer conditions of calmness, or the limited stories we tell ourselves, which may even be true as far as they go, but often just don't go very far compared to what might be if we were to tap into the larger dimensions of being available to us when we approach and befriend our own mind.

I Didn't Have a Moment to Catch My Breath

Are you stressed? Are you so busy getting to the future that the present is reduced to a means of getting there? Stress is caused by being "here" but wanting to be "there," or being in the present but wanting to be in the future. It's a split that tears you apart inside. To create and live with such an inner split is insane. The fact that everybody else is doing it doesn't make it any less insane.

Ekhart Tolle, *The Power of Now*

Tolle's assessment is as accurate a statement of psychological stress as any I have seen, the unfortunate endemic product of not accepting things as they are in the only moment any of us ever have in which to live.

But please be careful here. Acceptance doesn't, by any stretch of the imagination, mean passive resignation. Quite the opposite. It takes a huge amount of fortitude and motivation to accept what is—especially when you don't like it—and then work wisely and effectively as best you possibly can with the circumstances you find yourself in and with the resources at your disposal, both inner and outer, to mitigate, heal, redirect, and change what can be changed.

Approaching experience in this way is sometimes called "radical acceptance." Why? Because it goes to the root of things. It takes in and responds to how things actually are, underneath how they may appear to be and any preferences or aversion we might be harboring for how things "should" be or "should" work out. Recognizing and letting go of the stories we tell ourselves about how things should be and who or what is to blame because they are not that way is hugely difficult. But by adopting such a stance, we give ourselves the possibility of perceiving a deeper truth to things, one that often reveals how we might hold the circumstances and conditions we find ourselves in and act in ways that are wiser and more compassionate. Adopting a wiser and more accurate way of seeing and knowing and accepting of what is, the dynamics of what is are already different, and interesting shifts often follow in the wake of such a "rotation in consciousness," shifts that are only possible because you see a deeper truth that before you couldn't see because the story you were telling yourself, which usually isn't entirely true, if it is true at all, was too powerfully occluding your senses to let in anything else.

Yet, as a rule, even though in principle we may know better, we routinely succumb all the same to the incessant, often frantic, and unexamined busyness of thinking we have to get somewhere else *first* before we can rest; thinking we need to get certain things done to feel we have accomplished something *before* we can be happy... even as we are blaming our being busy and unhappy to a large extent on outside circumstances such as schedules and deadlines, employers' demands, the never-ending volumes of work to wade through and errands to run, or even on heavy traffic, which can so maddeningly thwart our desire to get where we want to when we want to.

Have you ever heard yourself say "I didn't have a moment to catch my breath!" when describing an episode during the day when you were going flat-out to get something done, so you could move on to something else, or get to the airport, or finally fall into bed?

We say it so facilely. "I didn't have a moment to catch my breath."

Linger with that one for a moment. Is it really true?

Or is it that we didn't think, or know to think that we actually could take a moment to orient, to ground ourselves in the body, to feel the breath and whatever tension and strain might be in both body and mind? If we can recognize what we are really doing and what we are really feeling in any given moment, we might be able to influence how we are *in relationship* to what is happening right in the very moment or string of moments in which things are unfolding. We could then choose to keep moving at the same pace or we might find that we could back off it a bit to good advantage and be more present and therefore perhaps ultimately more effective. We might even realize the folly of the way in which our desire to get it all done generates feeling chronically rushed or overwhelmed, which in turn makes it more likely that whatever doing we are engaged in is likely to suffer at least somewhat, if it does not wind up being severely compromised.

Then again, we may not feel we can stop in that moment, even if we consider it. We may feel that there is simply too much at stake. But we can always rush at least a bit more mindfully, thereby taking the edge off the moment of insanity we are caught up in and the "seriousness" of the situation, thereby shedding some of the stress of it all right in that moment. If, as we tell ourselves so frequently, there really is too much at stake to stop, then there is certainly too much at stake to risk being mindless and automatic.

By dropping in on ourselves, we can feel and inhabit the insanity of the intoxications we get caught up in. That gesture of mindfulness and lovingkindness can help us make longer-term choices to change when possible the way we set things up so that we can be less pressured. When our top priority is to inhabit the present moment regardless of the circumstances because we remember that it is all we have, and because we know that awareness is the most valuable resource we have to draw upon, then we have a chance to realign ourselves with sanity in a world that often seems mad, a world that would have it that insanity, in Tolle's sense, is sane and sanity insane, and also boring.

Such a realignment can happen in an instant. In fact, that is really the only time in which it can happen. All we need is to recognize the opportunity and remember that the world is not what we think it is and so we do not have to force some future outcome by betraying ourselves in the present. We can work with how things are now, however they are, as mindfully as possible.

That way, we might just learn how to catch our breath, and therefore our moments, and the rich possibilities of each one. Do you think we can risk being crazy enough to be that sane?

The Infidelity of Busyness

To commit oneself to too many projects, to want to help everyone in everything, is to succumb to the violence of modern times.

Thomas Merton

"I'm keeping myself busy." Lots of retired people say this kind of thing, probably to reassure themselves and others that they are not at loose ends and drifting into oblivion just because they aren't going to work every day, or receiving a paycheck.

One day I heard these words coming up from some deep crevice in my own mind and before I could stop them, they went right into the telephone.

"Wait a minute," I wanted to cry out. "What am I saying, and who the hell is saying this?" I am not keeping myself busy. If anything, I am attempting to keep myself unbusy, and finding that something of a full-time job. I moved away from pathological levels of busyness and doing, only to discover that it is not so easy to demur to either the outer or inner occasions that seem so attractive, so necessary, so important, so reasonable, and so containable—each considered separately—and yet, always wind up absorbing more energy than anticipated, making it difficult if not impossible to linger in the beauty of being in one place for months at a stretch, and living with a sustainable balance between right inward and right outward measure.

Saying "yes" to more things than we can actually manage to be present for with integrity and ease of being is in effect saying "no" to all those things and people and places we have already said "yes" to.

Why is that? Precisely because if we are overloaded to the point of being overwhelmed, it is likely that we will be so agitated, so distraught, so self-preoccupied, that we won't be able to meet anybody or any situation from a place of ease within the fullness of our own being in that moment, and that includes, most importantly, even an authentic meeting of ourselves and those we most care about. Perhaps we would do well to examine the impulses and seductions that drive us into such unfortunate circumstances.

Even if we tell ourselves that we are practicing mindfulness and embodying it as best we can from moment to moment, there are huge limitations and costs to disregarding or dismissing the possibility of a greater balance in the unfolding of things in our lives. When we set things up to make any real balance in our lives a virtual impossibility, we are evincing disloyalty to what we value most—which is literally what priorities are all about—and thus practicing, as poet and corporate advisor David Whyte so graphically and accurately articulates it, a kind of adultery, an infidelity. We may be betraying what is deepest and best in ourselves, and we may be betraying our relationships to others, even those we most love, and even our connectedness to places, to being at home where we are and fully in touch with what is most important and required in any moment. We might be losing touch, unknowingly, with our very relationship to the possibilities and the impossibilities of time.

Keeping such a radical view of our priorities in mind at key moments, it may be a lot easier to say "no" when our first impulse, and even our habit, is to say "yes."

Whyte frames this dilemma elegantly for us:

No matter what New Age gurus may say, we do not make our own reality. We have a modest part in it, depending on how alive we are to the way the currents and eddies of time are running. Reality is the conversation between ourselves and the never-ending productions of time. The closer we are to the source of the productions of time—that is, to the eternal—the more easily we understand the particular currents we must navigate on any given day. The river of time can suddenly turn, for instance, from a happy, easy flow to turmoil when, in the midst of everything, the boss asks us if we will take on a particular project that we know we cannot do with any sanity given all our present commitments; bereft of spaciousness, we say yes, trying to establish our identity through doing, afraid of the silence that might open in the presence of this figure of authority. Hounded by time, we feel hounded by others, but open to the spaciousness and silence, we can actually become fascinated by the silence that ensues from a pleasant but firm refusal. From the outside, our refusal looks like courage, but on the inside, it is simply representative of a healthy relationship with time. With regard to our marriage with time, to say yes would be the equivalent of promiscuity, of faithlessness and betrayal. Stress means we have committed adultery with regard to our marriage with time. If we want to understand the particulars of our reality, we must understand the way we conduct our daily relationship with the hours. In the hours is the secret to the workday, and in every workday the manner of our marriage to the hours and subsequently, our journey through the day, is crucial to the happiness we desire (*Crossing the Unknown Sea*).

One challenge of living mindfully is to be in touch with the natural rhythms of our own life unfolding, even if at times we feel far from them or we have lost touch with them altogether and find we have to listen afresh for those inner cadences and callings, with great tenderness and respect.

Our imagination about what may or may not happen in some other moment may go wild at times, out of desire or fear. In fact, that is bound to happen. But these intoxications and the anguish they bring with them can be counterbalanced and held in perspective by a wisdom that is slowly growing within us, a wisdom that emerges out of our fidelity to our own practice of mindfulness and to its embodiment in how we meet our moments and opportunities, writ large or small. It depends on keeping what is most important in mind, and recognizing our addiction to doing and thus, perhaps, to infidelity, or the fiction that we can balance it all, when the facts may be telling us that the costs are outweighing the benefits. It depends on remembering who we actually are, and keeping in mind, whatever we are engaged in doing or fantasize about missing out on—all of which is colored and distorted by our mindless perceptions and projections, mere fabrications of the mind—that whatever these preoccupations are, they pale in comparison to this moment that is.

*

One day you finally knew
what you had to do, and began,
though the voices around you
kept shouting
their bad advice—
though the whole house
began to tremble
and you felt the old tug
at your ankles.
"Mend my life!"
each voice cried.
But you didn't stop.
You knew what you had to do,
though the wind pried

with its stiff fingers
at the very foundations
though their melancholy
was terrible.
It was already late
enough, and a wild night,
and the road full of fallen
branches and stones.
But little by little,
as you left their voices behind,
the stars began to burn
through the sheets of clouds,
and there was a new voice,
which you slowly
recognized as your own,
that kept you company
as you strode deeper and deeper
into the world,
determined to do
the only thing you could do—
determined to save
the only life you could save.

MARY OLIVER, "The Journey"

Interrupting Ourselves

Whether it is to be better prepared to say no to your boss, or for being true to yourself in complex social situations with crosscurrents of expectation and conflicting interests, or to speak your truth to the voice of the "boss" that you may have internalized in your head and is now driving your life far more than you might want, or even want to admit, most of us could probably benefit from developing what behavior-change professionals call "communication skills" as a means of learning to convey, politely and with kindness, but all the same, firmly and assertively, how we are seeing a particular situation or more importantly, how we are feeling about it. Of course, before we can convey how we are actually feeling or seeing something, we have to be aware of that terrain within ourselves. And so often we aren't, or we are only partially aware of it. And that is particularly the case when we are feeling conflicted and torn, and all the options we can think of seem problematic, and maybe even too costly. We get caught up in those conflicted feelings, and are therefore, whether we know it or not, and whether we like it or not, *caught*.

Sometimes we can thread our way to clarity and mutual satisfaction in potentially difficult communications with others if we acknowledge and speak to the *feeling* coming from the other person, rather than being caught up in and perhaps reacting to the cerebral *content* of the conversation, which is hardly ever what such conversations are entirely about, and thus, at high risk for thinking we are entirely right and the other person entirely wrong, or wrongheaded.

Becoming even a little more mindful of how our conversations and communications unfold, and what kind of skills might be involved in navigating our way through them with greater awareness of what is really going on, inwardly and outwardly, in ourselves and with others, can be extremely revealing and humbling. To take just one common example, it may put us in touch with how frequently we are interrupted by others in the middle of our saying something, and it may also be able to help us identify effective ways of handling it when we are. Otherwise, and it is not a good feeling, especially if it becomes a pattern, we can wind up feeling like what we have to say doesn't count for the other person or in a group of people. We might wind up feeling disregarded, disrespected, undervalued, overrun, intimidated by certain people either at work or at home, and never effectively representing ourselves and how we see things and feel about things with clarity, conviction, and authenticity. And thus, the person, or family, or working group is potentially deprived of the benefit of our contribution, our creativity, our unique and potentially valuable vantage point. Meanwhile, we feel bad. And disempowered. And disregarded. And often angry at ourselves.

Ironically, the people who are doing the interrupting are usually completely unaware that they are not letting you finish what you were saying, and that they aren't really even listening to you. They might be surprised, even affronted, if you suggested that they tend to dominate in conversations, and are not good listeners.

They might soon forget it too, even after you have pointed it out, whether they were surprised by your assertion or not. That is because the habit of interrupting is so unconscious, so ingrained in us, so highly conditioned. To one degree or another, perhaps we have all been socialized to interrupt each other while talking. In a room full of argumentative men, it can sometimes look and feel like nothing less than rituals of virility and power, no matter what the topic up for discussion may be. Subtle or not-so-subtle racial, gender, age, and power differences and implicit biases can also come into play in this regard, leading to *dis*regard, and often worse. So it is helpful to ask ourselves: "Whose voice is not being heard enough or even at all in a family, in a meeting at work, or in the larger society?" And after asking that and reflecting on it inwardly, to hold whatever we realize from that inquiry in awareness, and perhaps with a bit more compassion and kindness than we might usually bring to our seeing of others, especially those who might look or be different from ourselves, and to at least attempt to see them in their fullness, in their humanness, or recognize in the moment how we might not be—and thus become an unconscious source of what are nowadays called microaggressions.

For the person who tends to be fairly out of touch with how much he or she interrupts others while they are speaking, which may include most of us at one time or another, it takes a lot of fortitude and presence of mind and openheartedness to take in and absorb such a pointing out of one's own automatic patterns of conversation, especially since, whether we know it or not, the interrupting is basically a display of self-centeredness, self-absorption, and sometimes unrecognized privilege that conveys that whatever I am impelled to say is more important, in this moment at least, and therefore can't wait, than any view or feeling that anybody else might want to express, no matter who they are and how much I care about them. A moment's reflection will reveal that such behavior can actually be a form of subtle or not-so-subtle violence, in that it can be harmful both to the individual you are interrupting, and therefore disregarding, and perhaps as well to the integrity of a collective process you are engaged in. It is a mark of character, once such a pattern has become conscious, to then be open to freeing yourself of it. It takes a great deal of mindfulness to accurately monitor your own behavior in the domain Buddhists refer to as *right speech*.

But if we resent being interrupted by others, and we also see how much we may also be doing it to others, perhaps we might do well to realize a whole other dimension of interrupting that we are ordinarily even more unaware of—and that is how much we interrupt ourselves!

We can readily catch this happening in our own meditation practice, especially our formal practice. Once we see it there, we are more likely to see it in our daily lives as well.

When we begin watching the unfolding of thoughts in the mind and sensations in the body in formal meditation practice, we rapidly discover that new events arise and distract our attention from what we were thinking or feeling just a moment before. Our experience of the moment is thereby interrupted, and often forgotten in the flight to the next thing that tweaks our hunger for novelty or our hair-trigger emotional reactivity. In this way, we can easily and unwittingly betray one experience, the one we are having, for another, hopefully a "better" one, without allowing the first actually to be held in awareness and complete itself. This is where the capacity for sustaining attention comes in.

Mindfulness practice does not only lead to our becoming more aware of this very strong tendency to interrupt ourselves, to distract ourselves and be diverted from what we are attending to in this moment, from what we might call our primary object or focus of attention. It also leads, of course, to training our attention to be more stable, more unwavering, less entrained into the interruptive and distracting energies of the thought stream and of transitory emotional states. In that way, over time, we are fashioning the instrument of our attention so that it is well anchored and stable and can, microscope-like, focus in on and discern what is unfolding beneath the surface of appearances and of our own unawareness at a much higher level of resolution and accuracy. Without this kind of stability in our awareness, we will continue to succumb to interrupting ourselves and not even know it.

And interrupting ourselves is really nothing less than subverting ourselves. It has a huge amount of dissipative energy in it, preventing us, if we are not careful, from ever really mobilizing the full repertoire of our strengths and creativity, and sensibilities. We can blunder along for decades in such patterns, missing what is right before us or within us, because we are always allowing the lenses through which we are looking to fog up. As a consequence, our own authenticity, our own authentic life direction can be missed, and we may wind up feeling truly lost and depleted without any inkling why. So, it can be profoundly useful and revealing to put those very instances in which we are diverted from our own greater purpose by our own self-generated interruptions—where we have nobody else we can blame for it but ourselves—to put them center stage in the field of our awareness when they arise, letting them become the object of our meditation practice in those very moments.

This interior habit of interrupting ourselves can also be seen at times in our outward behavior patterns when we are relating to others. That too can be a very valuable object of meditative awareness. Perhaps you have noticed occasions when, in talking with other family members, you don't let yourself complete a thought or a full sentence without blurting out the next thing that comes to mind, even if it is a huge nonsequitur, and another instance of not letting yourself complete a thought and thus, of interrupting yourself! We do the same in conversation with people outside the family. Our mind gets going and we stop attending. What is behind it may have too much momentum of its own in that moment for us to even hear what our own mind is saying, no less what anyone else is saying. That is when *we* start interrupting *them* as well as ourselves.

A little awareness can go a long way in this regard. But still, these unexamined habitual patterns of ours can carve deep ruts in the psyche from which it can be hard to extricate ourselves. It requires major intentionality to catch it happening, and then make sure we cease and desist. How will we ever know ourselves, how will we be able to listen to ourselves or understand ourselves if we keep on interrupting ourselves without even knowing it?

And how will we ever be present for someone else if we refuse to

listen and we keep finishing other people's sentences (because we tac-
itly assume, with considerable arrogance, if you stop and think about
it, that we know better than they do what they are trying to say), or if
we wind up unconsciously blurting out whatever is dominating in our
own mind at the moment, even though it may have no direct relationship to what was just said?

The quality of our relationships with others, to say nothing of the
quality of our relationship with ourselves, can suffer greatly if we do
not bring some modicum of awareness to this arena. This is something I try to keep in mind every single day. It is easy to talk endlessly
about it. It is not so easy to enact.

Filling Up All Our Moments

In response to those same chaotic agitations in the mind, often stemming from transient sense impressions, that lead us to interrupt ourselves so much of the time in addition to our propensity for interrupting others, we also tend to keep filling up all our moments so we won't be idle or bored or have to deal with stillness.

We go from one thing to the next all day long, even when we are working. It might be checking your messages or e-mail, texting or instagraming or snapchatting, reading the newspaper, picking up a magazine, channel surfing on TV or YouTube, watching a movie on Amazon or Netflix, calling people, going to the refrigerator, turning on the radio as soon as we get in the car, running errands, compulsively cleaning up our living space, reading in bed, saying mindless things that are irrelevant in the moment but simply reflect the quasi-random thoughts that continually plague us. All these and more totally normal ways of spending our time, at least some of them necessary to keep our lives going and take care of what needs taking care of, can also be ways to keep ourselves perpetually distracted from being fully in the moment, fully awake.

If we start to pay attention to these impulses as they arise, we may find that we are virtually (all puns intended) addicted to distracting ourselves, so habitually do we float through our moments and fill them up with activity and stuff without landing in them.

We fill up our time and then wonder where it all went. We divert ourselves in all these ways, like a river can be diverted, then wonder—in those times when everything comes into some kind of greater focus for a moment or two—where we are in our lives and why we feel so far from the mark, so far from our deepest aspirations, from contentment, from peace, from really being at home within ourselves and in deep connection with others. We may wonder in such moments where our lives are taking us or why things aren't somehow better and more fulfilling than they are, have a bad night or two, and then fall back into our habitual diversions, in large measure because they make us feel better in the short run, and they pass the time that otherwise might feel interminable, empty, scary.

Maybe, when it comes right down to it, we actually are afraid of having time, even as we complain that we never have enough of it. Maybe we are afraid of what might happen if we stopped interrupting ourselves or we stopped filling up all our moments, and instead just settled into now, even for a few breaths. Maybe we have exactly the right amount of time and we have forgotten how to be in wise relationship to it.

What would it be like to settle into your own body, into a sense of just being alive, even for a few moments, or say, five minutes at the end of the day, lying in bed or just sitting around in the evening, or at the beginning of the day, before you even get out of bed? What would that be like? You can find out of course, just by dropping in on yourself and purposely not filling the present moment up with anything, especially anxieties about the future and everything you "should" be getting done, or resentment about what has already transpired and hasn't gone exactly as you desired. You can try being aware of it if such emotions do arise and start to churn away inside of you, especially in the form of impatience, anger, fear, worry, resentment, or sadness. You can play with seeing what it is like to linger with such feelings and just breathe with them for a tad longer than you are likely to think you can possibly stand it. And in such moments, you can always ask yourself whether your awareness of discomfort or agitation is itself uncomfortable or agitated. And, even when you are not agitated, you can always remember, say, when you are taking a shower to check and see if you are actually in the shower, or whether your mind is off someplace else filling itself up and forgetting to drop in on the here and the now—and feeling the water on your skin.

Even on vacation, we can fill up all our time seeking desperately to have a good time, only to wonder where it all went, or to come home feeling vaguely dissatisfied. We have the photos to prove we were there, but were we really? The "postcard from the edge" reads:

"Having a great time. Wish I were here."

Someone once used that line in describing his experience at the end of a seven-day MBSR professional training retreat. It got a huge laugh because we were all so aware of how much the mind checks out by filling itself up. It is humbling to watch how much that happens, even when practicing meditation. Actually, especially when practicing meditation, because, of course, we see it much more clearly when we are watching the mind so carefully. Remember Basho (see Book 1, "Hearing"):

> *Even in Kyoto—*
> *Hearing the cuckoo's cry—*
> *I long for Kyoto.*

Even in solitude, even in pristine wilderness, it is easy to fill the time with longing, with reveries, with chores or various preoccupations, or with the desire for "sightseeing." All these fluctuations in the mind and body may separate us from nature or from the matter at hand and have us anticipating what will be coming next, or caught up in memories or desires. The sightseeing mind may make it impossible to really see anything of interest or importance, or even the sights that you are privileged to see. You are always on the lookout for a better moment, a better view, a better experience. If you saw the bear cub, you weren't close enough. Or perhaps you only saw the fluke of the whale, but missed seeing the whole of its body out of the water when it breeched.

In a moment filled with such thoughts, we may miss entirely the *sound* of the whale breeching, or of a fox barking. And we may miss the silence too, even the silence of pristine wilderness, because the mind is always too filled with its own noise to detect it. In this way, we can easily miss the present moment beyond the thought, beyond all compulsive need to be doing, to be someplace else, to seek something new and exciting, no matter how compelling to that acquisitive aspect of the mind, no matter how much we can rationalize our desires in terms of our momentary happiness or unhappiness.

We could even ask at such moments, "Who is it that needs something new and exciting?" and "What exactly is 'excitement' anyway?" And how will it end?

Lying back and watching clouds, bathing in birdsong or the desert breeze, feeling the air around the body, the heat coming off canyon walls, the play of light on stone; or feeling the muscles on the back of your neck tighten as you try to find a parking place downtown in a snowstorm when you are already late for an appointment, whatever is offering itself to you in the place where you find yourself—wilderness, metropolis, or suburb—why reject it and seek elsewhere for excitation and entertainment and distraction when life is always unfolding here and now, and there is no place better and no other time? What sense is there in self-distraction, when, like the diverted river or stream, it shunts us out of our lives and fills our perfect moments and our beautiful minds, difficult as they might be at times, with just what is not needed?

Could you possibly be here, wherever you are? With whatever is happening? Now?

If so, you might find that you are already having a great time, greater than you knew. Perhaps, when all is said and done, you are simply comfortably ensconced at home...in yourself, independent of circumstances, wherever you are.

As one of the many one-liners putting meditation practice in wry perspective that circulate on the Internet has it:

Wherever you go, there you are. Your luggage is another story.

*

A mother was teaching her young child to tell time. They reviewed together: "When the hands of the clock are together like this, both pointing straight up, it is twelve o'clock, time for lunch. When they make a straight line, like this, it is six o'clock, time for dinner. When they are like this, it is nine o'clock, time to go to your play group. When they are like this it is three o'clock, time for your bath."

The child responded: "And Mommy, where is plenty of time?"

*

What if we all have plenty of time, but then we forget? Mindfulness has everything to do with remembering, reconnecting, and coming back to the availability of our lives in any and every moment. But however many moments we may have, they don't go on forever. The law of impermanence is ever-present and hard to fathom. So why not seize the moments we have, and string them together into plenty of time, plenty of time for being awake with what is, for taking care of what needs taking care of, and for knowing how to ski that edge so that we are at home in our own skin more of the time, rather than blasting through some of our moments to get to better ones later on? This is it. Just this.

Just this.

Attaining Place

In California one winter, there was a moment during walking meditation on a deck off the meditation hall—which looks out from on high above a stream descending in a ravine between two significant hills where, on my left as I faced southeast, a small jungle in the crease between the hills flourishes and immediately contiguous with that, in front of me, bare Marin hill-edge sloping down left to right at forty-five degrees, beyond it an uninterrupted vista across the valley to distant hills—when I experienced a kind of visceral seizure through all the sense gates at once that I was in California.

Of course, I knew I was in California before that, having flown in to the San Francisco airport a few days earlier. But in that moment on the deck, I "attained" California. California was realized, confirmed, and revealed. It immediately brought to life boyhood memories, sights and smells and feelings (felt in the way one feels a place when one is six or seven and it is not one's native place and it is very different from what one knew before). In that moment, California, or at least that place, that micro-environment called Spirit Rock Meditation Center in Marin County, with all its locally unique qualities of earth and air and water and life, down to its characteristic vegetation and the din of mating sounds from the frogs in the stream, was seen, was smelled, was heard, tasted, felt, and known.

A faint cool moistness off the early morning mountain
Wraps my face like a muffler
And wafts enticingly into receptive apertures.
Walking out of the dining room
I lift up mine eyes (the archaic wording arrives as if revealed
and seems right for such an archetypal moment, just as in the Psalms)
Unto the hills,
Golden in the soft morning light.

In the days before that moment on the deck, I guess I was only in my idea of California. It took a while to arrive completely. Attaining a place can happen anywhere, at any time, if you manage to be present without your usual filters. Otherwise, you might only be in your idea of the place, whether it be California, or Paris, or a Caribbean vacation spot, or your office for that matter, and never attain it. That postcard from the edge may very well apply: "Wish I were here." But you are! But you are!

Another oft-told tale carries a similar reminder. African tribesmen were hired to guide a U.S. television crew with a lot of equipment through the jungle to the city. Because of time pressures, the news people insisted on a rapid pace that they kept up for days. Finally, within a day's walk of the destination, the porters refused to go any farther despite all pleas, exhortations, and promises. The TV people pointed out imploringly that they were almost there, that one last effort would complete the journey. But the tribesmen were adamant. The reason? They had traveled at such an unnatural pace that they needed to stop for a time and let their souls catch up with their bodies.

For only when we fully arrive and are present, outside of thinking and fully in our senses, can we attain a place. Perhaps this is the ongoing puzzle, challenge, and conundrum of our lives. Can we, when all is said and done, at "the end of all our exploring...arrive where we started and know the place for the first time"? T. S. Eliot phrases it as an affirmation. We shall. We shall!

We shall not cease from exploration
And the end of all our exploring
Will be to arrive where we started
And know the place for the first time.
Through the unknown, remembered gate
When the last of earth left to discover
Is that which was the beginning;
At the source of the longest river
The voice of the hidden waterfall
And the children in the apple-tree
Not known, because not looked for
But heard, half-heard, in the stillness
Between two waves of the sea.

T. S. ELIOT, from "Little Gidding,"
Four Quartets

But what would it mean to arrive where you started and know the place for the first time? And what would it take? When shall we realize it? And do we know that we already have what it takes, and are it? Do we know that we are already there... I mean here?

Eliot's final stanza of *Four Quartets* continues without any break in the meter, line, or rhythm:

Quick now, here, now, always—
A condition of complete simplicity
(Costing not less than everything)
And all shall be well and
All manner of thing shall be well
When the tongues of flame are in-folded
Into the crowned knot of fire
And the fire and the rose are one.

"A condition of complete simplicity." Where do you suppose we could find it?

"Costing not less than everything." The stakes are that high. This really is the adventure of a lifetime. And in parentheses, no less!

"And all shall be well." Perhaps all is already well...perfectly what it is. Perfectly as it is. Here. Now. Arriving.

Attaining here. Attaining now. And knowing here and now for the first time, moment by moment by moment.

You Can't Get There from Here

There is more to arriving where we started and knowing the place for the first time than meets the eye. For one, we are at risk of it never happening. So many things can get in the way, especially the way we think, or the notions we cling to without ever examining. Attaining place, or view, any place, any authentic view, requires openness. Ultimately, it does require a condition of complete simplicity, so that we can see what is available to be seen and know what is available to be known, both of which are impossible if we persist, especially without knowing it, in only seeing through the so-often-limiting lenses of our own ideas, opinions, and experiences, however wonderful and erudite they may be.

Radical openness to what we have not yet experienced does cost not less than everything. Sometimes we don't want to pay the price, so attached are we to having it our way, or so conditioned we are to thinking we know what our way might be, when of course, we are always newcomers, each and every one of us, continually approaching the horizon of the just-beyond-the-familiar, the unknown. And underscore *always*, whether we know it in any moment or not. In this territory, trust in one's deepest intuition, even when it runs against the dominant grain of conventional thinking, is paramount to both creativity and discovery, and ultimately, to liberation from our own attachments and blindnesses.

If we are indeed continually learning, then, painful and difficult as it may sometimes be, and however much by fits and starts, ultimately we will be compelled by experience to look at and transcend the boundaries of our own tacit assumptions—often a product of our professional training, in addition to the conditioning we are entrained into from early childhood—and the patterns of perception and thought we fall into so easily because of familiarity and comfort, and because they work so well in certain circumstances. Such habit-driven mind patterns, implicit biases, and tacit assumptions can at times ensnare us into modes of thinking and understanding that preclude orthogonal perspectives, try as we might to wrap our mind around novel perspectives intellectually. This is true for all of us at times, no matter how proficient or insightful or learned we might be. For me, it is a continual lesson in humility and non-attachment, and it is a hard one, one that I fail at over and over again. Ultimately, it is the lesson that everything in life is practice, not just the things we like or the situations that go our way. It is a perpetual invitation to trust one's intuition and experience and remain open to not knowing, even, or especially, in the face of our own blindnesses and shortcomings.

At such times, something else entirely is required, something utterly brave and daring, because it involves surrendering terrain we are comfortable and familiar with for the terrain of the unfamiliar, for what is not yet known, beyond the horizon of what we can see but that we just might intuit somehow as being important to visit. This is likely to be very scary, and not so easy to do. In fact, nothing is more difficult.

The following is an account of how a new field developed within cognitive therapy, a development that required that radical shifts be made in the way "psychological treatment" was conceived. I tell it because mindfulness has become increasingly popular within many relatively traditional psychological circles. This is in part due to MBSR, and primarily as a result of the work recounted below, which has come to be known as mindfulness-based cognitive therapy, or MBCT. MBCT, along with other mindfulness-based approaches, such as DBT (dialectical behavior therapy), ACT (acceptance and commitment therapy), Mindful Self-Compassion (MSC), and various so-called "mindfulness-informed" psychotherapies, have already transformed the landscape of psychotherapy and psychology. But MBCT led the way when it came to grounding psychological therapy in formal and intensive meditation practice.

The growing interest in and enthusiasm for mindfulness is due in large measure, I would say, to an emerging hunger for authenticity and clarity and peace within ourselves, a hunger that the world is now displaying on so many different fronts. I see it as a very positive emergence, potentially a hugely healing emergence in our world. Yet, as mindfulness becomes more popular, inevitably first as merely a concept, it is very easy for it to become divorced from its grounding in practice and thus from its healing, transformative, and liberative potential. Because it is on its face such a good and compelling *idea* to be more present in one's life and less reactive and judgmental, some professionals naturally assume that it can merely be grasped intellectually and then taught to others that way, as a concept, and that that can be done without a solid grounding in one's own personal practice. But without the practice, no matter how clever or articulate or sensitive or therapeutic what one is offering may be, it just isn't mindfulness, or dharma. For it is the practice itself* that provides entry into the orthogonal space, beyond the conventional views we are usually so caught up in. As we have seen over and over again (see Books 1 and 2), it is the practice itself that is the vehicle for our coming to our senses and waking up to the full spectrum of what is and what might be possible.

In 1993, as recounted in their book, *Mindfulness-Based Cognitive Therapy for Depression*, Drs. Zindel Segal, Mark Williams, and John Teasdale, distinguished colleagues in clinical psychology and cognitive science from, respectively, Toronto, North Wales (then Oxford), and Cambridge, England, came to visit the Stress Reduction Clinic for the first time. They had initially heard of our work from Marsha

---

* See Book 2, *Falling Awake*, Part 2 for explicit practice instructions and descriptions.

Linehan, a behavior therapist who had developed a well-researched and highly successful approach known as Dialectical Behavior Therapy, or DBT, for treating people with a condition known as borderline personality disorder. Marsha herself is an accomplished researcher as well as a skilled therapist, long-time student of Zen, and now a Zen teacher. DBT incorporates the spirit and principles of mindfulness, as well as whatever degree of formal practice is possible for the people who are plagued by this particularly trying constellation of afflictions, including high rates of suicide and suicide attempts.

By that time, Zindel and Mark and John had been collaborating as a team for eighteen months to develop a new form of cognitive therapy to prevent recurrence in major depressive disorder, a debilitating condition that is very prevalent in the world and that can interfere enormously with the ability to work, sleep, eat, and enjoy once pleasurable activities. For compelling theoretical reasons as well as for important and very practical clinical reasons, they had decided that, at that juncture, a logical and potentially critical extension of their work would be to introduce a group-based training program including mindfulness meditation and its applications to daily living, along the lines of MBSR, for people suffering with this condition.

In particular, their idea was to explore the effects of mindfulness as an attention-regulation strategy in synergy with more traditional aspects of cognitive therapy to address in a potentially novel way a very serious problem associated with major depression, namely that people who have been successfully treated with antidepressants and are therefore no longer clinically depressed still suffer high rates of relapse, in other words, are at high risk of falling back into depression once their treatments come to an end.

For a number of reasons, they suspected that a group-based mindfulness training approach, blended with appropriate cognitive therapy procedures, which for the most part are used in individual therapy with people rather than in groups, might help them to address more effectively the strong tendency of people who suffer from major depression to fall into thought-streams of depressive rumination, even after they have been successfully treated for the acute episode of depression and are no longer are depressed. This kind of rumination can itself trigger and then amplify depressive thinking and tip the person into an increasingly downward spiral, leading to full-blown relapse.

Their reasoning for wanting to explore the possible use of mindfulness to deal with these negative ruminative tendencies was theory-based and extremely insightful. Their reasoning led them to suspect that mindfulness might provide an effective framework for (1) teaching their patients what they referred to in their specialized terminology as "decentering skills" (meaning the ability to step back and observe in a less self-identified way one's own thinking as it is occurring, seeing one's thoughts simply as thoughts, as events in the field of awareness, rather than as necessarily accurate reflections of reality or of oneself, whatever their content might be); (2) training them to recognize when their mood was deteriorating so that they could initiate the inward stance of decentering; and (3) again in the words they used in a technical, theoretical report, making use of "techniques that would take up limited resources in channels of information processing that normally sustained ruminative thought/affect cycles."

My colleagues and I could sense from the very beginning of our conversation that afternoon that their individual and collective motivations for embarking on the proposed project were suffused with both compassion for people suffering from this extremely prevalent worldwide illness and a wonderful enthusiasm for expanding the scope of their scientific understanding of and clinical approaches to the knotty dilemma of high relapse rates.

Of the three, only John had had any formal meditation experience at that time. He had a long-standing meditation practice and some experience using it successfully with individual clients, and held a deep conviction of the potential therapeutic value of cultivating non-judgmental and accepting states of mind, through mindfulness, for people with recurrent depression. But it was also clear that Mark and

Zindel, by their own admission, didn't have much of a practical sense of what they were getting into on the mindfulness side. They had no experience with formal meditation practice and no particular interest in it. It was their interest in the whole question of what they were calling "attentional control" and its potential usefulness as perhaps an effective vehicle for enhancing decentering in a clinical outpatient group setting that had stimulated their willingness to take a look at MBSR. The three of them had planned to develop an agreed-upon treatment, test it by having each of them conduct programs for patients in their respective countries, and combine the results they each obtained as part of a research study on the effectiveness of this approach.

Of course, central to the cultivation of mindfulness is the systematic practice of recognizing and observing thoughts from moment to moment as events in the field of awareness with stable and discerning attention, and as best one can, intentionally making an ongoing and systematic effort to attend to them without either judging them or getting caught up in their content, as well as recognizing those moments when one does indeed inevitably get caught in either of those ways and not judging oneself for that.

Cognitive therapy, too, focuses on identifying and observing thoughts, but more discursively, and within a problem-solving framework that assesses their content as accurate or inaccurate and attempts to substitute more accurate and health-enhancing thoughts for those with a more inaccurate and potentially self-defeating content. Our visitors had been led by various lines of evidence and reasoning to suspect that it was actually the moment-to-moment identification of thoughts in the mind *as thoughts*, rather than a preoccupation with their content, which was a key pathway through which cognitive therapy was having its demonstrated therapeutic effects on depressive relapse in the individual treatment of patients. If so, they reasoned, then the mindfulness approach, which features a much more robust and sustained development of attention and a more disciplined formal practice of attending to thoughts as thoughts than does cognitive therapy, might be particularly useful for dealing with recurrent negative rumination. Thus, their initial intention was to see if it might not be possible to combine mindfulness with cognitive therapy. They suspected that the mindfulness practice might address in a more direct and effective way the three key issues mentioned above, namely "decentering," sensitivity to early warning signs of a negative mood shift, and intentionally cultivating attention in ways that would "take up space" in certain information-processing channels in the mind that would otherwise be vulnerable to defaulting to depressive rumination.

Combining mindfulness as an attention-focusing and decentering strategy with a more conventional problem-solving cognitive therapy approach looks feasible theoretically, but from the very beginning, they had significant doubts about how effective mindfulness would be in dealing with resistance, or with any difficult emotions or crises if and when they arose out of the practice itself or in the course of their patients' lives. Their thinking at that first meeting was that their therapeutic expertise would take care of those issues if they arose.

Adding or combining different intervention elements in a therapeutic process is a fairly common practice in clinical psychology, and it makes sense if all you are doing is introducing one more method or technique for attention regulation, or to enhance relaxation, or for cultivating insight into a broad spectrum of approaches that are all being deployed in the service of a successful therapy. The added module or technique either "works" for someone or it doesn't. So it is not out of the ordinary for professionals to think of mindfulness along similar lines, as a potentially important technique or module that they can "plug in" to a therapy framework to serve a particular and well-defined function, while the rest of the therapy is taken care of by the other elements. In the case of our visitors, they had already intuited that the mindfulness would require a radical shift away from the standard perspective of cognitive therapy, and that combing the two while giving each its full due might be hugely challenging, if it were possible at all. And we, from our vantage point, were concerned that without across-the-board training and experience in mindfulness meditation among all three of them, they would inevitably find themselves falling back on their perspective and skills as highly trained therapists, and thus unable to represent and feature the full spectrum and depth of the meditation practice in its own right. We were concerned that this approach might result in the meditation practice winding up *de facto* functioning at best in that "modular" way, as one "technique" in combination with a whole array of other more conventional therapeutic approaches, in spite of their best intentions.

As soon as we sat down to talk together and heard what they were hoping to do, we tried to emphasize that mindfulness is an orthogonal universe. It does not lend itself well to limited modular applications, at least as long as one maintains a conventional framework of seeing it as a "technique" that people can use and get good at and which will "work" for certain things but might not for other things. After all, mindfulness meditation isn't merely an attention-regulating clinical strategy, even though it can dramatically deepen both stability of attention and insight. Nor it is a relaxation technique, even though it can induce deep states of relaxation and feelings of peace and well-being. Nor is it a cognitive-therapy technique to solve problems by restructuring your thought patterns or your relationship to specific emotions or mood states, even though it can have transformative effects on a person's relationship to habitual thought patterns and to emotional reactivity and absorbing moods. Moreover, it is not exclusively oriented to the thinking process, independent of emotions, emotional turmoil, and emotional reactions. Nor is it independent of what is going on in the body and in the wider world. In mindfulness practice, these domains and everything else that happens within the experiencing of one's various states of mind are all embraced as one seamless whole, as different aspects of one's personhood and lived experience.

We also emphasized that mindfulness is not really a therapy at all. Its primary aim is not to fix a person or correct a specific problem. From our perspective, weird as it may have sounded to anyone who had no familiarity with meditation from the inside—and we admitted that it might have sounded *very* weird, especially in the professional context of adopting it as a clinical intervention where everything is understandably oriented toward getting good outcomes—we explained that mindfulness as a formal meditation practice and as a way of living one's life involves non-doing more than it involves doing anything, that it invites the exploration and cultivation of what we call *the domain of being*. Any change that may occur comes out of the rotation in consciousness that frequently stems from the shift from the doing mode to the being mode, rather than by intervening to fix a problem or bring about a specific outcome, as is so much the case in cognitive therapy. Nevertheless, it was clear, we said, from our experience in the Stress Reduction Clinic with people with a wide range of medical disorders, as well as those suffering from panic and anxiety disorders, that if practiced wholeheartedly *as a way of being*, mindfulness can and does lead over relatively short periods of time, such as the eight weeks of MBSR, to profound health outcomes for a wide range of people and problems, including significant symptom reduction, more effective dealing with emotional reactivity under stressful conditions, and insight into deeper dimensions of being and into old and confining habits of thinking and feeling.

If mindfulness really is a way of being, a way of seeing, sensing, and feeling, rather than merely a technique, then we stressed, if they wanted to incorporate it into a treatment for relapse prevention for major depression and really have their patients engage in the formal meditation practices wholeheartedly and with some degree of discipline and constancy, there would be no getting around having to set up an approach that would allow and encourage mindfulness to be cultivated with a non-striving orientation, for its own sake, so to speak. It would have to be taught within a context of ongoing practice, inquiry, and dialogue, and in its own language, a language that, everybody in the room was well aware, is very different from that of cognitive therapy. The practice would have to be presented on its own terms, as a radical non-doing, inviting a counterintuitive inward stance of acceptance and opening rather than fixing or problem solving, and in such a way that, hopefully, it would be experienced by prospective participants as a new and perhaps friendlier and more self-compassionate way of being in one's body and embracing all of one's thoughts and feelings with acceptance without either judging them or trying to substitute one thought or pattern of thoughts for another.

In other words, mindfulness could not possibly be combined with cognitive therapy without denaturing its very essence, unless all these considerations were taken into account. If they hoped for it to be of any value, from our point of view, they would have to feature mindfulness training and practice as the core organizing principle for the entire enterprise, and thus, mindfulness would have to constitute the core of what was employed when faced with difficult emotions and challenging circumstances. Anything less was likely to result in the effort becoming a caricature of what mindfulness really is, putting it at risk of becoming denatured and thereby losing its intrinsic power and the richness of its multi-textured and nuanced dimensions.*

That was quite a message for us to be delivering and for them to be taking in at a first encounter. It was not at all clear to us that they had, as a group, realized the full downstream implications of adopting that orientation for themselves as individuals and as a team, and for their patients. Since they were so open and congenial, we felt comfortable being frank and direct with them about how we saw things.

But there was another issue as well. They had originally, and very understandably, thought it would be possible to have their patients

---

* You might think that our psoriasis study would suggest that it is possible to just "plug in" a guided meditation audio program and get a good result without any kind of group participation at all, or any instruction or feedback beyond the tape itself. But that protocol was adapted for a very specialized and limited purpose under unique circumstances, and is not particularly relevant to a group-based program led by an instructor oriented toward people at high risk for depressive relapse.

learn to meditate and practice merely by having them use our guided meditation audio programs on a regular basis, including during the classroom sessions themselves. Although John Teasdale, as we noted, had a long-standing interest in meditation and a personal meditation practice, at that time he did not have any hands-on experience teaching meditation to a group of people, a role that is quite daunting and sobering for anyone to undertake under any circumstances, even after one has been practicing and teaching meditation for years.

It soon became clear that they had not, as a team, seriously considered the possibility that, in order to do what they hoped to do, each one of them would have to not only be practicing the meditation himself, but also guiding and instructing his patients in the various practices during the classes proper, based on his own direct, first-person experience with practice, whatever audio guidance they decided to assign for daily homework between the classes. When we brought up the fact that, from our perspective, it was not going to be very effective, if even possible, to recommend that others meditate without having an ongoing meditation practice oneself—how, for instance, would you be able to answer your patients' questions about their meditative experiences if you had not had similar experiences yourself? For Mark and Zindel at least, this was certainly an unexpected turn of events.

The orientation of asking others to do something you don't actually engage in yourself (and so, in the case of meditation at least, would have no direct, first-person experience of), as contrasted with an orientation that calls for undertaking to practice yourself along with your patients, underscores something of the fundamental differences in thinking that sometimes arise between conventional therapeutic treatment approaches in psychology—where methods are employed in the service of achieving specific desirable therapeutic ends—and training in meditation—where the practice is engaged in non-instrumentally, (see Book 1, "Two Ways to Think about Meditation: The Instrumental and the Non-Instrumental") as a way of being for its own sake rather than simply as an instrumental technique to achieve a more desirable state or view.

Moreover, there is a strong professional ethic among therapists that suggests keeping an airtight separation between one's own private personal needs, interests, and engagements, whatever they may be, and the needs of one's patients. Yet here we were suggesting that in order to really understand the practice of mindfulness and the effects it might have on one's patients, one would have to engage in it wholeheartedly oneself, which amounts to agreeing to go on an adventure, the nature of which is, to a large degree, unpredictable, and that cannot possibly be strictly professional, in the narrow sense, since one is presumably growing as a person oneself in the process. That is not to say that the highest ethical standards of professional conduct and awareness of appropriate boundaries would not be adhered to and honored, merely that one's view of oneself as a therapist would have to stretch to accommodate the role of meditation teacher in its full embodiment, quite a tall order.

But even speaking in the most basic practical terms, how would it be possible to share and explore mindfulness practice with one's patients if one were not cultivating it oneself? The moment-to-moment familiarity with the nowscape that comes with practice, the systematically cultivated firsthand intimacy with one's own mind, including all its activities, resistances, distractions, and with one's own body and everything it goes through in response to one's own thoughts and moods would not be part of the daily repertoire of two of the instructors, even as they would be asking just that intimacy and effort of their patients, or should be if they hoped to make full use of the meditation practice's potential for healing and transformation. Were that the case, there would be no reliable platform upon which they could stand in relationship to the patients' meditative experiences, no authentic reservoir of experience from which to answer the patients' very real questions about their practice and respond skillfully to their feelings about it, to their difficulties and their insights in bringing it into their daily lives.

My colleagues and I were happy to be having this conversation with them, happy that professionals of their stature were drawn to our work and were looking for a way to adapt it to their own field and their own clinical interests. This was exactly what we hoped would happen, for mindfulness to become a growing positive force in medicine and health care and beyond. But, as I sat there listening that afternoon, I found myself sensing a deep gulf between our frames of reference, as if our vocabularies and ways of speaking about mindfulness were somehow missing a way to connect, even though I suspected there might be one. At the same time, their openness and authenticity and caring were palpable. I found myself pondering how to possibly communicate our radically different way of seeing the challenge they were posing themselves in a way that would be helpful, without it seeming that we were merely clinging obtusely to a narrow and parochial point of view because we were comfortable with it or were feeling threatened by their suggestions or perspective. I felt impelled to somehow try to make clear what I saw as the core problem with what they were proposing, while at the same time, honoring the evident fact that both their intuition and motivation were clearly right on target.

We had reached a lull in our conversation, and had fallen into silence for a few moments, overcome, I guess, by the enormity of what we were touching together and the sense of the gulf between us. Finally, I broke the silence. "You know," I began, "there is a colloquial expression used on occasion by people living along the rugged Maine seacoast. When asked for directions by tourists who flock there in the summer, they are famous for replying, 'Oh, you can't get there from here.' I find myself feeling more and more that way about what you are proposing."

It was not to deflate their idea or motivation, which I am certainly not doing justice to but which you can read for yourself in their own vivid account of this encounter and of their subsequent visits with us. Or maybe it was just a tiny bit, in part to see how they would respond, to test their resolve to find a way to "combine" mindfulness and cognitive therapy that we could collectively agree upon was commensurate with the breadth and depth of mindfulness practice. What I was trying to say was that in order to understand mindfulness, never mind the intricacies of how to integrate it into their clinical work, it wouldn't work for only one of them to be practicing if they were all going to be delivering the intervention. They would all have to practice the meditation formally and informally, and not just a tad for the taste of it or for the sake of appearances, or even to experience for themselves what they were asking of their patients; but wholeheartedly, for themselves, following the same overriding principle we adhere to in MBSR, namely that we do not ask anything of our patients that we do not ask at least as much everyday of ourselves.

But how, I wondered, was this trio of eminent scientist/clinicians, deeply grounded in their cognitive therapy models and vocabulary, only one with firsthand experience of meditation practice, going to find a way to agree on a course of action in their work together? And as members of a team, how was each of them individually going to put aside whatever professional reservations he might be harboring about taking on not only the *practice* of meditation, but also the *teaching* of meditation? How were Mark and Zindel, the two with no previous interest or experience in meditation, each individually going to step sufficiently outside of a framework that had come from years of a certain kind of training and professionalism, even to want to take on the practice for themselves, and to do so perhaps first out of curiosity but later, perhaps, out of some deeper motive rather than just because we were saying it couldn't really be understood any other way? Would their motivation as individuals and as a team to do this work and follow their deepest intuitions carry them that far from their original expectations, conceptualizations, and reservations? Especially since it would probably mean giving up their specialized cognitive therapy vocabulary when teaching their patients, shifting from a therapist mode to more of a mindfulness-instructor mode, as well as deliberately putting aside for a time at least their clinical viewpoints, ideas, and conceptual models of how the mind works.

Instead, we were suggesting that they each move personally into the practice in a systematic and disciplined way, and watch the unfolding activity of their own minds and bodies, taking whatever emerged on its own terms for a time rather than being concerned with immediately relating it to theories of attentional control, or to their patients' minds and the problems of depressive relapse. Of course, some of that would be unavoidable, the inevitable content of the thought stream. And of course, in the long run, some kind of synthesis would be necessary, inevitable, and very desirable. We were not denying that. But could they intentionally suspend their usual frame of reference, their cognitive coordinate system, for a while, and simply practice watching their own minds and bodies?

I hardly expected that they would be inclined to undertake such an adventure individually and collectively. Yet that, to our way of seeing, was the bare minimum of what it would take to do what they wanted to do and have it be authentic. Without it, there was simply no way to get "there" from "here." Ironically, if they were to find a way to let go of the particular lenses they were using, not that that would be easy, they would discover that the "there" that they wanted to get to was already "here." All that would be required would be to shed one set of lenses for a while and bring a fresh set, or what we might call the "non-lenses" of original mind, to bear on what is unfolding moment by moment within one's own experience, that is, through bare, clear, non-judgmental, non-reactive, non-conceptual attention. Since none of them had experience teaching meditation in a group setting, that aspect of it, as a practice in its own right, in addition to developing their own personal meditation practices, would take some time and a lot of deepening. All in all, they would be making one hell of an investment if they decided to pursue it, with no guarantee that it would be successful. They could only come to such a decision individually and together as a team, and of course, only for their own reasons. But what they were looking at was, from our perspective, an enormous leap into the unknown.

Remarkably, they came to do just that, and not because we said so, but because they were intrigued by what we were saying, and found it jibed with the intuitions and motivations that had brought them to visit in the first place, and even more so, with their experiences with their patients upon returning home. They piloted their ideas into a first attempt at a clinical intervention, as recounted in their book,* and, more often than not, indeed did find themselves falling back on their cognitive therapy instincts and skills when strong emotions and other problems arose in the classroom, rather than addressing them as part of the meditation practice itself. That initiatory experience teaching mindfulness brought them back to the Stress Reduction Clinic to sit in on more classes to get a better sense of just what was going on in MBSR, and to observe different MBSR teachers and study what the instructors were actually doing and how they were doing it at different stages of the process. Sometime during that second visit, Mark and Zindel decided that, like John, they would take up the regular daily practice of mindfulness meditation themselves.

It became very clear from later exchanges that they had thrown themselves into the practice wholeheartedly, not primarily as professionals but as people, and had to face and deal with their various professional discomforts and reservations. By their own account, it was painful, it was difficult, it brought up a good deal of doubt and struggle at times. But each of them in his own way either deepened or embraced and persevered with regular practice and worked at bringing to it a motivation based on curiosity and self-compassion, in addition to the

---

* Segal, Z. V., Williams, J. M. G., and Teasdale, J. D. *Mindfulness-Based Cognitive Therapy for Depression*, 2nd edition, Guildford, NY, 2013. See in particular the introduction, in which they recount their perspective on these visits with extraordinary personal candor and scientific acumen.

desire to help others suffering the afflictions of depressive illness. They got a good deal of encouragement and moral support from everybody at the Center for Mindfulness as we grew to love them and respect them, and came to appreciate the magnitude and depth of the innovation they were bringing to cognitive therapy and their skill as scientists and clinicians, to say nothing of what a pleasure it was to be with them. And those friendships have only grown deeper over the years.

As a result of their personal explorations and scientific investigations, John and Mark and Zindel have made major contributions over the intervening years, both singly and together, in the treatment of depressive relapse, none of which I imagine would have come about had they not had the courage, as a team, to suspend their own professional framework for a time and, each in his own way, simply drop into stillness and watch the unfolding of their own direct experience from moment to moment, doing nothing less than using their own lives and experiences as the laboratory for understanding, in a different, more direct, and complementary way, their own minds, as well as the minds of their patients.

That they undertook to do this together is a marvel. That they persevered over days, weeks, months, and years, through thick and thin, even more of one. To me, their attitude and tenacity were embodied proof, not that we needed any, that status and ego-attachment were not fundamental motivators in their lives. They did not appear to be either personally or professionally defensive about the path they were embarking on, although some concerns were expressed, with frequent smiles, about what their professional colleagues might think once it became known that they were actually practicing and teaching meditation. They were clearly open to learning and expanding their framework for approaching the mind and, something that the cognitive therapy tradition does not emphasize, the body as well. And their book does a radically courageous and imaginative thing: It tells the story of the development of mindfulness-based cognitive therapy from the point of view of their own personal experience and learning curves, something that is almost never done in an academic textbook. Taking this tack gives readers a deep sense of what is actually involved in authentically pursuing a path that brings together two very different but powerful approaches to understanding the mind and catalyzing healing from suffering. As a consequence, and of course, also because their scientific study of the effects of their work was so well done and the results sufficiently impressive, many of their colleagues have found their book and the work it describes not only scientifically compelling but also inspiring. Its publication, along with an ongoing series of scientific papers describing their work, has led to a remarkable surge of interest in mindfulness and its applications in the field of clinical psychology. It also led to the founding of the Oxford Center for Mindfulness at the University of Oxford in 2008 by Mark and his colleagues, itself a remarkable achievement.

More recently, John and Mark and Zindel published another equally elegant book, this time a do-it-yourself workbook for their patients, for people who are suffering from major depressive disorder and wish to have an effective resource for in their self-directed efforts to apply mindfulness for dealing with and freeing themselves from the deep ruts of depressive rumination.*

I think that each of them would acknowledge, if pressed, that their views of the mind and the body and what might be possible for their patients have grown more nuanced, more sensitive, more insightful, and perhaps more optimistic, perhaps with even a greater faith in what people are capable of, because of their own engagement with the practice and teaching of meditation, and because of the range of effects they have observed among the people who have experienced their program now over many years. If true, this is not something that they got from us, but rather from their own deepening experiences of

---

* Teasdale, J., Williams, M., and Segal, Z. *The Mindful Way Workbook: An Eight-Week Program to Free Yourself from Depression and Emotional Distress*, Guilford, New York, 2014.

mindfulness practice. Over the many years of our collaboration and friendship, we have learned from them at least as much as they have learned from us, and in the process, we all continue to enjoy the mystery of our work together and separately, and our love for the relationships and adventures it has spawned. And those adventures continue.

Their work has contributed in major ways to the building of a bridge between two worlds that, until the past decade or so, almost never talked to each other, the world of clinical psychology and the world of meditation practice, and underneath that, of dharma. Traffic in both directions across this bridge is now contributing to refining insight and understanding in both worlds. What is more, their ongoing studies and scientific insights into the nature of emotion and how it can be regulated through attention to reduce suffering and liberate people from the dark shadows of depression is contributing in large measure to the continuing development and spread of mindfulness-based approaches to healing, approaches grounded in the firm understanding that they need to be rooted in the meditation practice itself rather than merely in mindfulness as a *concept*.

OVERWHELMED

One day, I had a phone conversation with a professor of religion prior to a visit to his campus to meet with a faculty group about developing a contemplative curriculum in the university for undergraduates. In the course of the conversation, he told me that he was extraordinarily busy, what with all his committee responsibilities on top of his teaching and scholarship, travel, and raising young children at home.

For some reason, my first reaction was to laugh and tease him a bit about it. Then I realized that it wasn't so funny, certainly not for him. It was diagnostic, a telltale sign of our age, and I found myself feeling sad, and a little disappointed. Somehow, deep in the recesses of my psyche, I had been harboring an archetype of the Ivy League professor, especially a scholar of Asian studies and longtime meditation practitioner, leading a quiet and peaceful life on an idyllic campus. I shared with him that if he were talking about the medical school, or the law school, or the business school, or even the biology department, I wouldn't have been at all surprised. But the religion department! The humanities!?

In saying it, I realized how compartmentalized my own mind was. There was still a romantic memory trace of a former time, perhaps when I was in college in the early sixties, when things really did seem slow and leisurely, with life unfolding on a more human scale and at a rate that wasn't conducive to a sense of perpetual overwhelm. Of course, that is, leaving out the violence of segregation in the South, the Cuban missile crisis, and the like, but even the missile crisis seemed to unfold in slow motion, trapped as we were into being help-less spectators at what could have turned into "the end of the world."

Now though, our inner, first-person experience of things happen-ing is so speeded up that we hardly know what is happening to us or around us, either individually or collectively. Like the proverbial frog put into water and then gradually heated, we often don't realize how fast and furious and hot things have become for us until we experience that we are already getting scalded; or, in the frog's case, winding up dead without having attempted to leap out, as he would have, they say, if dropped into hot water to begin with. Speed itself has snuck up on us. It has gradually become a way of life we are now addicted to and complacent with without even knowing it. We have been entrained into perpetual acceleration, with ever-increasing expectations to get more done quicker and sooner, to process endless amounts of infor-mation, both the desirable and that which we are merely bombarded by or addicted to, to be instantly gratified, even if it is just by the speed at which our computer boots up in the morning, if we ever shut it off, or by how fast we can get on the Internet. As we have seen and know deep in our hearts, we are running so fast to keep up with our schedules and to get things done and to acquire what we want and run from what we don't want that a lot of the time it feels as if we are run-ning on empty, with no time to catch our breath, or just be still with no agenda, or even pause to be happy with what we have achieved or attained already, or to feel our pain and sadness.

To have even a chance of maintaining our sanity in the current era, we may have to become intimate with stillness, every one of us. Stillness and periods of quietude may no longer be luxuries, if they ever seemed to be, nor experiences only suited to monks and nuns who have renounced the worldly life, or to adventurers in wilderness, or vacationers in national parks. I am not talking about leisure time. I am talking about non-doing. About spending deep time resting in pure wakefulness, outside of time, with the mind spacious and open.

If it is healing for us when faced with life-threatening and chronic diseases, how can it not be healing for us in the face of the dis-ease of feeling totally and chronically overwhelmed and bereft, that our lives are somehow unfolding faster than the human nervous system and psyche are able to manage well.

I once was asked to lead a mindfulness workshop at a business conference in Chicago. About fifty people in suits showed up. I opened our time together by suggesting that we simply sit together for a few minutes with no instructions and with no agenda. I suggested that we let go of whatever expectations and stories we were bringing into the room about the workshop and why we were there (after all, something brought them there, no one was in the room by accident), put down our coffee cups and newspapers (this was before smart phones!), and just take a few minutes to allow ourselves to feel how things were for us in that moment, however they were. A few people started crying.

In the conversation afterward, I asked what the tears were about. One executive said, "I never ever do anything without an agenda." Heads nodded in agreement. Just the words, "let's sit without an agenda," were liberating, releasing dammed-up feelings of grief they didn't know they had.

It is possible that each and every one of us, in our own way, may be starving for no-agenda time, for non-doing, for stillness, beyond even the concept of meditation and the concept of me doing either something or nothing (such as the thought "I am meditating now"). I am not talking about distracting ourselves with our phone, the newspaper, or snacking, or conversing with others or with ourselves, or daydreaming either. I am talking of being aware, resting in being, in cognizance itself, beyond thought, in being the knowing and the not-knowing that awareness already is. In what Soen Sa Nim (see Book 1, Part 1) termed, in his own inimitable way, "don't know mind."

DIALOGUES AND DISCUSSIONS

Learning how to listen to and value the perspective of others, especially if you are aversive, if not allergic, to their views and positions
and methods, is an important part of healing divisions that can fester
and turn toxic, as we see happening so much in the world, nowadays.
Otherwise, we just live within our own self-confirming comfort bub-
bles and bemoan those "others" who are the source of all bad things.

In certain circles within the world of business and the world of
dharma, certainly within the MBSR community, we speak of *dialogue* as
the outer counterpart to the inward cultivation of moment-to-moment
non-judgmental awareness, or mindfulness. Just as in the practice of
mindfulness, in dialogue, we attend to whatever "voices" are arising in
the mindspace and the nowspace (See Book 2, Part 1) of the meeting
itself, hearing, feeling, touching, tasting, knowing the full spectrum
of each arising, its lingering, its passing away, and whatever imprint or
aftermath it leaves in the next moment, without judgment or reaction
(or with an awareness of judging and reacting if they do arise, which
of course they will at times). In this way, we can give ourselves over
to being in conversation with others in dialogue. Just as we need to
feel open and safe in our own meditation practice, so we need to create enough openness and safety and spaciousness of heart for people
in a meeting to feel safe in speaking their minds and from their hearts
without having to worry about being judged by others. No one needs

to dominate in a dialogue, and indeed, it would cease being a dialogue at that point, if one person or group attempted to control it. We watch the arising of and listen to the voicing of ideas, opinions, thoughts, and feelings, and drink them all in in a spirit of deep inquiry and intentionality, much as we do in resting in awareness in formal meditation practice, allowing it all to be treated as equally valid, to be seen, heard, and known without the usual editing, censoring, vetting, criticizing, or rejecting. Surprisingly, a feeling of a collective intelligence that seems to reside in the group itself but is not localized in any one person often emerges under such conditions, and with it a deeper insight, or shared recognition of what direction to go in as a direct consequence of such intentional spaciousness, openheartedness, and deep listening.

This is often sadly not the case when we are in meetings with colleagues at work, or in the domain of politics, or even in our own family, where contending agendas, well-fortified positions, and self-righteousness may dominate discourse. The norm is to have *discussions* rather than *dialogues*. We discuss things endlessly in meetings. We have agendas, we plan for things to happen, we decide on a path and then execute our strategies and action plans. But often, there are hidden agendas and major power differentials between people in such discussions that remain unspoken, often even unknown by the participants, and which do a certain kind of violence within the process itself when the orthogonal dimension is not present or valued.

So it may be of value to bring mindfulness to the whole dimension of how we conduct ourselves in meetings with others, especially when the stakes are high, things need to get done, and the group needs to function coherently together, even within a diversity of sometimes strongly held views and opinions and positions. Whether it is General Motors developing its strategic plan for the future, or diplomatic deliberations, or peace talks, bringing mindfulness to the table, along with the elements of what some people call non-violent communication, becomes critical if there is a hope that a new level of

understanding and accord might be reached that will further learning, growing, healing, mutual understanding, and the transforming
of potential and possibility into actuality.

Learning to listen and participate in conversation with others is
the heart of such healing, and of true communication and growing. It
is an embodiment of relationality and mutual regard. In true dialogue,
no one's views, opinions, and feelings in a group are invalid, no matter what the power differentials. They only turn toxic or degrade the
potential for "progress" to come out of "process" if they are discounted
or not attended to at all. It can be healing simply to be heard, to be met,
to be seen, to be known. And out of such meetings, true orthogonal
possibilities can emerge, just as can happen through openly meeting
oneself in silence and stillness.

For these reasons, I find it useful to distinguish between the terms
"dialogue" and "discussion" and be mindful about their uses based on
my relationship to and intentions for particular gatherings. I am not
advocating striking the word "discussion" from our discourse, but
to keep in mind what purpose discussions serve and how they often
unfold in actuality, especially in the absence of a greater embrace of
awareness and intentionality by the entire group. The word is defined
as (1) to speak with others about, to talk over; and (2) to examine or
consider (a subject) in speech or writing. It comes from Middle English *discussen*, to examine, from Anglo-Norman *discusser*, from Latin
discussus, past participle of *discutere*—to break up (dis = apart; cussus
= to shake, to strike). The deep meaning is to shake apart. The Indo-
European root *kwet*, to shake or to strike, is also the root of concus-
sion, percussion, and succussion. You get the drift.

"Dialogue," on the other hand, stems from the Greek *dialogos*,
conversation, from *dialektos*, to speak. *Dia* means "between," and the
Indo-European root *leg*, or *lektos*, means to speak. Thus, dialogue carries the meaning of speaking between or among in conversation, and
often, as in the Socratic dialogues, in a spirit of deeply investigating

together through open inquiry. The quality of the relational space is the key to emergences and openings.

Not a bad way to walk into a nine o'clock meeting, even if no one else suspects. But with time, groups can intentionally adopt this kind of approach to their common work, and in doing so, the work becomes a much more shared, and often far more creative and productive enterprise, or should I say, adventure? Imagine if governing bodies took this approach.

SITTING ON THE BENCH

I don't know many professions where the operative verb in the job description is "to sit," but one of them is judges. Judges "sit" on the bench, and in sitting up there, for it is an elevated seat in most courtrooms, they bear witness to a steady parading of the worst things human beings do to one another and to themselves. And they are supposed to bear witness dispassionately, wisely, while overseeing and regulating and ruling on the unfolding of all the evidence and narratives marshaled for and against the particular charges levied against the defendant or defendants. The judge creates and maintains the container that ideally allows the jury, if it is a jury trial, to drink in the relevant facts and arguments in a measured, discerning way. Only then is the jury to come to a decision through considered deliberation as peers of the defendant or defendants (in criminal cases) or as peers of the plaintiff and defendant (in civil cases), in other words, as the regular folks that they are, hauled in at random for jury duty, and carrying within them in these unusual (for them) life circumstances, the repository of whatever wisdom and fairness is immanent in our hearts and therefore in our legal system—as participants in the right it accords to all citizens, the right to a trial before an impartial jury of peers.

I was once invited to conduct an eight-week MBSR program for a group of Massachusetts district court judges. I soon learned that stress is a huge occupational hazard for judges. Day after day, week after week, they preside over and drink in the horrors and, eventually, the tedium of a continuous stream of graphic evidence of the unfortunate consequences of human greed, hatred, ignorance, and inattention, writ small or large, depending on the case. On top of that, their every word in the courtroom is taken down and becomes public record. Everything they say is at risk of being picked up by the media and quoted out of context. If they slip up for one second, they can be open to huge potential criticism from the press and public, so there is a tendency to say as little as possible. There is also the natural danger that at any time, they could be caught napping (because the cases can become monotonous and boring, especially after you have seen an endless stream of similar ones).

All this being the case, judges naturally tend to feel somewhat cautious, in part because of professional standards of judicial restraint, and also lest they wind up looking foolish. They also have to come up with opinions and verdicts in non-jury cases, and these can be another source of stress, as they inevitably satisfy one party and not the other, or satisfy no one. And at times, their decisions can create major political fallout that only compounds their stress, whether they are elected to office or appointed for life. What is more, they obviously cannot and would not want to share with their families each night how their day went in any detail. But unless they have some highly effective way to be transparent to it and rest in true equanimity and wisdom, they have nevertheless perhaps absorbed a modicum of toxicity that day, just by showing up for work and hearing the evidence and the arguments.

To top it all off, as a rule, they have not been taught to sit, even though that is the operative verb in their job description. So, learning how to sit within the context of MBSR seemed karmically perfect for these district court judges, and we had a great time practicing together over the eight weeks of the program. For the first time for most of them, they had a forum for talking about their feelings fairly openly with their peers in a context that was emotionally safe and protected, since it took place at the hospital, away from the courthouse and all judicial trappings, and since their stress was being addressed within the larger context of mindfulness practice and the cultivation of different ways of working with it creatively in their unique circumstances.

A few months after I had worked with the judges, I was at a party at a friend's house in Western Massachusetts, where I met a young lawyer, Tom Lesser, who, as it turned out, happened to be a practitioner of Buddhist meditation. He told me the following story.

He was one of the defense lawyers in a famous case in Massachusetts that was being tried in Amherst in 1987. It was known as the Amy Carter, Abbie Hoffman trial. Amy Carter was the daughter of former president Jimmy Carter. Her improbable codefendant was Abbie Hoffman, the famous 1960s political activist and "Yippie" leader who, as one of the Chicago Seven, was a defendant in one of the most publicized, cantankerous, and controversial trials in U.S. history. Hoffman had subsequently gone underground to escape the law on a drug charge, and had had plastic surgery to disguise his face. For a number of years, he had managed to lead a respectable, even public life under an alias in a suburban community in upper New York State as an environmental activist. In fact, disguised as mild-mannered citizen activist Barry Freed, he had been appointed to a federal environmental commission by President Carter, had testified before a U.S. Senate committee, and had received a citation from the governor of New York at the time for his environmental work and community organizing on the St. Lawrence River.

In any event, Amy Carter and Abbie Hoffman, no longer underground, had teamed up with a number of other people in November of 1986 to protest CIA recruitment on the flagship campus of the University of Massachusetts, in Amherst. About one hundred of them were arrested for trespassing and disturbing the peace, and fifteen were ultimately brought to trial, as they had wished to be from the very beginning for their act of civil disobedience. The case became known in the press as "the CIA on trial." The defense put expert witnesses on the stand, from a former U.S. attorney general to a former CIA agent—and convinced a jury of six, using a strategy known as the "necessity defense" or "competing harms doctrine," that the civil laws the defendants had broken were minor compared to the criminal acts being committed by the CIA, specifically to fund an illegal war in Nicaragua through the Iran-Contra affair. Prominent witnesses testified that the CIA's actions were in violation of national and international law, and that the defendants had no effective alternative but to act in the way that they did in order to put a stop to the ongoing criminal actions of the CIA in violation of the express wishes of Congress. In the end, Carter and Hoffman and their codefendants were acquitted. The case got a good deal of national publicity.

As a member of the defense team, Tom was in the courtroom when the judge gave what is known as a "pre-charge" to the jury after it was finally selected but before any evidence was presented, something that was quite out of the ordinary in and of itself. Generally, jurors are not told how to look at a case until it is finished, after all the evidence has been presented. So imagine Tom's astonishment when he hears the judge say, addressing the jury (and here I am now quoting verbatim from the official court transcript, although when Tom told it to me, he told it to me in his own words): "It is important that you understand the elements of the case. It is also important that you pay attention with the terminology that I became aware of some time ago of mindful [sic] meditation. Mindful meditation is a process by which you pay attention from moment to moment to moment. It is also important that you maintain an open mind, that you make no determination on this case until all the evidence has been submitted for your consideration."

Being a longtime practitioner of mindfulness, Tom said he practically fell off his chair when he heard those words. The judge was giving mindfulness instructions to the jury!

Some time after the trial ended, Tom went to visit the judge in chambers to find out where he had learned about mindfulness and meditation. In Tom's recollection, the judge, Richard Connon, said something to the effect of: "Well, I had just taken this stress reduction program for judges at the medical school at UMass. During the course, Jon Kabat-Zinn talked about how important it was to look at things moment by moment by moment. Well, that was just a stunning concept to me. I had thought about looking at things moment by moment, but there was just something radically different about watching events unfold moment by moment by moment—the idea that attention could be that ongoing and continuous was just amazing to me. Now, that is also exactly what you want a jury to do. So it just seemed like a good idea to tell the jury how to pay attention in that way in order to help it to listen non-judgmentally."

Judge Connon brought up the mindfulness instructions again, right before the closing arguments in the case. Quoting once more verbatim from the trial transcript: "I ask you now to pay particular attention to the closing arguments but also to pay very close attention to my instructions. You will recall to mind that I used the term back then that I will use again today, in making reference to mindful meditation, all right? I don't want you to go to sleep, although I think it is rather impossible in those chairs, but I want you to pay attention from moment to moment to moment. It is important. It is important because the standards of our justice are such that you today will exercise the rights that we have under the Constitution, both the Federal Constitution, the Constitution of the United States, and the Constitution of the Commonwealth of Massachusetts, and it is very important because you represent every citizen in this country."

Maybe juries should routinely be given mindfulness instructions before every trial. Here are some generic words that any judge could use to cover the bases briefly and comprehensively, without ever using the word "meditation": "I want you to listen to what will be presented in this courtroom with total attention. You may find it helpful to sit in a posture that embodies dignity and presence, and to stay in touch with the feeling of your breath moving in and out of your body as you listen to the evidence. Be aware of the tendency for your mind to jump to conclusions before all the evidence has been presented and the final arguments made. As best you can, continually try to suspend judgment and simply witness with your full being everything that is being presented in the courtroom moment by moment by moment. If you find your mind wandering a lot, you can always bring it back to your breathing and to what you are hearing, over and over again if necessary. When the presentation of evidence is complete, then it will be your turn to deliberate together as a jury and come to a decision. But not before."

You Crazy!

One night, back in the early Seventies, I gave the public Wednesday-evening talk at the Cambridge Zen Center. Then Soen Sa Nim, who had been sitting next to me the whole time, answered questions. It was his way of training his students to become teachers.

The very first question came from a young man halfway back in the audience, on the right side of the room, who, as he asked the question (I forget entirely what the import of it was) demonstrated a degree of confusion that caused a ripple of concern and curiosity to pass through the audience. Necks craned as discreetly as possible to get a look at who was speaking.

Soen Sa Nim gazed at this young man for a long time, peering over the rims of his glasses. Utter silence in the room. He massaged the top of his shaven head as he continued gazing at him. Then, with his hand still rubbing his head, still peering over his glasses, with his body tilted slightly forward toward the speaker from his position sitting on the floor, Soen Sa Nim said, cutting to the chase as usual: "You crazy!"

Sitting next to him, I gasped, as did the rest of the room. In an instant, the tension rose by several orders of magnitude. I wanted to lean over and whisper in his ear: "Listen, Soen Sa Nim, when somebody is really crazy, it's not such a good idea to say it in public like that. Go easy on the poor guy, for god's sake." I was mortified.

All that transpired in my mind and probably the minds of

everybody else in the room in one moment. The reverberations of what he had just said were hanging in the air.

But he wasn't finished.

After a silence that seemed forever but was in actuality only a few seconds, Soen Sa Nim finished: "...but [another long pause]...you not crazy ennuffff."

Everybody breathed a sigh of relief and a feeling of lightness spread through the room.

It may have been beneficial for this young man to receive such a message at that particular moment and in that particular way from the likes of someone of Soen Sa Nim's lineage and imposing stature. At the time, it actually felt both compassionate and skillful, given the circumstances. I have no idea whether it was useful for him or not. I hope it was. I can't recall if Soen Sa Nim followed up with this man or not, but one thing was very clear about him—he never gave up on anybody.

I like to think that Soen Sa Nim was saying that we need to dare to be sane, to take on our craziness unabashedly and hold it with compassion, to face it, name it, and in doing so, be bigger than it, no longer caught by it, and therefore, intimately in touch with our wholeness, not only sane, but saner than sane. Especially when what passes for sane these days on the world stage is often madness itself—with truth often the first casualty.

PHASE CHANGES

If our true nature is, indeed, wholeness, why do we feel fragmented so much of the time? How can this be understood?

Here's an analogy that might be helpful. From physics and chemistry, we know that water can manifest in a number of different forms depending on the temperature and pressure. At sea level, it is a liquid at room temperature. It becomes a gas and boils off if heated to 100 degrees C (212°F). And it freezes into a solid if cooled to below 0 degrees (32°F). But whatever form it takes, it is still water.

These transitions between solid, liquid, and gas are known as *phase changes*, because the water changes from one form, or phase, to another. In the different phases, the water molecules, the H_2O molecules, have very different relationships to one another... that is why ice is hard and why water from the tap can flow and can assume the shape of whatever container it is in, and why steam or water vapor fills the entire volume it is placed in. Yet, whether it is in the form of a solid, a liquid, or a gas, it is always H_2O, just assuming different forms depending on the circumstances (of temperature and pressure—remember that on Mount Everest, water boils at a temperature far below 100 degrees C because the air pressure is so low; that is why it is hard to cook things at high altitude... boiling water is not very hot, the way it is at sea level).

We could say that H_2O is the fundamental or true nature of water (its original essence). Depending on changing conditions, it can exist as a solid, a liquid, or as a gas. In each of those forms, it will be characterized by very different properties. In other words, its outward appearance and "feel" will be different, and it will behave differently.

It is the same with the mind and the body. The mind and body too can go through what feel like phase changes as conditions change. The changing conditions can create pressures of one kind or another, or alleviate them. Changing conditions can heat things up or cool things down emotionally, cognitively, somatically, socially, even spiritually. We call these various changing conditions that require us to adapt one way or another "stressors," and we refer to our experience of those changes, especially if we do not respond adaptively to them, as "stress."

Reacting to stressful situations, whether in the outer landscape or in the inner landscape, our minds and bodies can change instantly as the impact makes itself felt. We might become paralyzed or "frozen" with fear, for instance. We have all experienced that at one time or another. The mind can also be frozen, say, in a particular idea or opinion, or in resentment and hurt. It can quickly become rigid, unyielding, cold, and this frozenness manifests in ingrained patterns of thought, emotion, and behavior. Or it can heat up with agitation, confusion, anxiety, bewilderment, kind of like steam. We even speak of blowing off steam. No doubt we've all had some experience of both extremes. Or the mind can feel somewhere in between, more like slush, not quite ice, not quite water, just plain messy and unclear.

At other times, when conditions are different, if we are free of pressure and things don't feel like they are heating us up to the point of boiling, or freezing us to the point of contraction and rigidity, the mind can be quite spacious, like a gas, expanding infinitely and subsuming whatever unfolds within it, or like water, flowing freely, unimpeded over and around boulders and other obstacles in our path.

Sometimes these phase changes happen spontaneously, as a result of changing causes, conditions, and circumstances in the outer landscape of our lives, whether it be work, family, the larger society, and/or economic or political upheavals. But much of the time, they also stem from our own self-generated agitations and reactions within the inner landscape. They stem from our unexamined habits of mind, through which we can unfortunately lock in to particular long-standing patterns of thinking, feeling, and seeing (or not seeing) that keep us rigid and frozen. In such situations, whether triggered by outer conditions or inner events, we are often unable to remember and recognize our true nature, which is not limited to or bound by the frozen state or any other state, but is really the underlying, H_2O-like essence that allows us to assume many different states of mind and body, and therefore respond with greater wisdom and effectiveness in the face of the various outer challenges and inner fluctuations of mind and body that we may be faced with in any moment, and indeed, that we are actually faced with to one degree or another in every moment.

It is mindfulness that can help us thaw from the frozen condition into the freer condition of spaciousness, and to realize that even spaciousness is not our true nature, but rather just one more manifestation of it.

We might say that our true nature is our ability to know, the innate awareness that can hold any and all states and phase changes and know that they are only manifestations of our underlying wholeness that transcends form and phases of any kind, whether it be ice, liquid, or steam, or the Zen teacher Joko Beck's whirlpools (See Book 1, "Emptiness"). Ultimately, it is not the stressors that throw things one way or another, although it is so easy to blame outer conditions or our inner state of mind for our dis-ease or for our despair or dysfunctional behavior. Rather, it is our *attachment* to them, our impulse to hang on and cling to them that locks us in, first by not recognizing the true nature of the arising events, which as we have seen is fundamentally empty, and second, by resisting, struggling, contracting, blaming, hating, and trying to force a reality that we don't like to change in a direction we would consider more gratifying or pleasant or more secure for us—without first recognizing the deep structure of what is happening and the full range of our options for being in wise relationship to it.

If awareness itself is our true nature, then abiding in awareness liberates us from getting stuck in any state of body or mind, thought or emotion, no matter how bad the circumstances may be or appear to be. But when we are locked in the ice, for instance, we don't even believe in the possibility of liquid water, nor do we remember that our true nature is beyond any of the various forms that it can assume. One moment of remembering can liberate us from a lifetime of habitual contraction, because we no longer take one phase or another as who we are or what is most fundamental.

The twelfth-century Korean Zen Master Chinul put it this way:

Although we know that a frozen pond is entirely water, the sun's heat is necessary to melt it. Although we awaken to the fact that an ordinary person is Buddha, the power of dharma is necessary to make it permeate our cultivation. When the pond has melted, the water flows freely and can be used for irrigation and cleaning.

That melting, that free-flowing, expansive awareness in an inter-embedded universe feels a lot like love—the sun's heat releasing the waters of both mind and heart. It is available to us in any and every moment, if we remember what is most fundamental.

Neuroscientists like to speak of various "states" that the brain or nervous system can be subject to or fall into, patterns of activity that have a self-similar if dynamic identifying characteristic. So it is not surprising that it is all too easy for the word "state" to somehow creep into being associated with mindfulness, as if there were one particular mindful "state." There is not. If we were going to associate the word state with mindfulness, it seems to me that it would be to say that mindfulness is the state (or set) containing all possible states. But then, it would be pure awareness, or put differently, H_2O. So as you keep up your meditation practice, it is critical from the beginning to remind yourself that you are not trying to achieve or attain a particular state, or feeling, or insight of any kind—and to notice it when you discover that you are very much indeed trying to get someplace else or feel something more desirable than what is already unfolding. What you are engaged in is inhabiting the awareness that embraces and recognizes non-conceptually the *phase* of whatever state you may find yourself in, whether it is the mental or bodily equivalent of ice, water, or steam, and remembering that you are already, in all cases, the metaphorical equivalent of H_2O.

You Make, You Have

Soen Sa Nim, in the very same lineage as Chinul, only eight centuries later, was fond of saying "You make problem, you have problem." What he meant was simple, and unbelievably relevant. There are really no such things as problems. The concept "problem" is just that, a concept, an overlay, an interpretation of a situation. Thinking turns situations into problems.

Problems are fine for math or physics homework, but in life there are actually no problems, only situations that require a response, hopefully adequate to the circumstances and the challenges each one presents. And that does usually involve some kind of accurate assessment and even instinctive or well-thought-out calculations of probabilities. Situation means a circumstance that presents itself as it is, in the immediacy of what it is, of things as they are. But too often, when we turn situations into problems, then we shift our whole psychological orientation over to having a problem, and this orientation can narrow our ways of seeing just when we most need to stay open and creative and not get caught in the heaviness of having "a problem," or worse, a "big problem," which also instantly makes for a more reified "me" or "us" that is having it.

One day, my daughter reported a big puff of flame out of the oven just as she was beginning to bake her delicious almond-flour banana bread. After that, the oven went off and wouldn't go back on. I check the burners on top of the stove and see that they do not light when I turn the knob, and the igniter doesn't do its usual clicking. Same for the oven. Since we had problems with the "stove" not too long before that required a repair person to visit, I say we will have to call the repair people. Too bad, the banana bread will have to wait.

Then my wife, Myla, says, "What about checking the circuit breaker?" In the moment she says it, I know that is what is causing this problem. Why didn't I think of that? I'm the one who is supposed to think of that, to know that. I go downstairs and sure enough, the circuit breaker for the stove is tripped. I reset it, and voilà, the oven is working again.

In one instant, my mind had turned what was going on into a problem with the stove itself and so didn't allow for the possibility that emerged in Myla's mind. Instead of staying open to the situation, my mind had turned it into the problem we had had before rather than the situation that we are having now. The hasty misdiagnosis precluded any more clear thinking, in that moment at least.

So the challenge of each and every moment is, can we approach things in such a way that we act appropriately in each situation, moment by moment by moment, whether what we are dealing with is pleasant, unpleasant, or neutral, familiar or unfamiliar, known or unknown? And can we do so even as the thinking mind wants to and frequently does, out of habit, automatically turn what is arising into "a problem," perhaps even misperceiving it at the same time, as I did, and the small "I" gets into the act and turns it into a dilemma or even a melodrama—the story of me and my problem and how it is going, or not going?

After a while, "You make problem, you have problem" got condensed into simply "You make, you have," and thus expanded to include any "construction project" of the mind, big or small. It was one of Soen Sa Nim's many ways of teaching us that thinking itself is a fabrication (from the Latin *fabricari*, to make something). It places a screen between us and direct experience. He was suggesting that it might be good to become aware of it each time it happened so that we wouldn't unknowingly get caught up in it and lose touch with direct perception and direct knowing. Clear thinking, analytical thinking, can be extremely useful and powerful. But often our thinking is not so clear; and it can completely obscure the domain of direct experience, and other ways of knowing that are not mediated by thought.

I was enchanted to discover decades later that, in a similar vein, the Tibetans speak of "non-fabrication" as a fundamental attribute of what they call original pure mind or "the great natural perfection" (Dzogchen). We might say, and confirm for ourselves just by watching our minds, that what all meditative traditions refer to as the untrained mind is always fabricating ideas and opinions, views and problems, just as Soen Sa Nim was suggesting. This "idling" of the mind is sometimes referred to as "proliferation" in meditation texts because thoughts, fantasies, and daydreams, all with their emotional ripples, proliferate endlessly. This proliferation, this incessant fabrication is virtually invisible to a mind unfamiliar with watching itself non-judgmentally. We would have no idea that it is even happening. This is exactly what William James was bemoaning in his statement about an education that would help us to recognize and bring back a wandering attention, and we could say, synonymously, a wandering mind, over and over again. (See Book 1, Part 2).

The mind that has some experience with training in mindfulness still experiences proliferation and fabrication because they are simply an aspect of the mind's nature. But with training and the cultivation of greater stability of mind, and the development of some degree of equanimity and insight, such activity is recognized and held differently. It is not uncommon to see proliferation and fabrications of mind in increasingly subtle ways, along with increasingly subtle forms of clinging and grasping. The grosser manifestations of proliferation and fabrication may not go away, but their oscillations tend to damp down considerably if they are not constantly fed and reacted to; and, at times, they can attenuate completely and simply dissolve away.

How does this come about? When we cultivate mindfulness, it is the mindfulness itself, as it becomes more stable and refined, that detects fabrication as fabrication *as it is occurring.* Our awareness chooses not to feed it by getting reflexively and mindlessly caught up in the habit of attaching to it and thus spinning out proliferating stories about it. When approached in this way, the fabrications of the mind in the form of thoughts and feelings, ideas and opinions, are more likely to be recognized rapidly for what they are, insubstantial, evanescent formations, simply events in the field of awareness that arise and inevitably pass away, like clouds in the sky or like writing on water—both images rendering so accurately and so picturesquely the incessant dance of the mind and the transience of its contents.

If we can bring an attitude of non-fabrication to our practice on the meditation cushion and off of it, on the yoga mat and off it, the mind's spacious, knowing, and compassionate essence is more available to us. How might we do that? First of all through the intention to not make anything, even the thought that you are meditating, or that now you will be more aware of fabrications...those too are fabrications, although perhaps more skillful ones. So are the endless narratives that we are so accustomed to telling ourselves about our experience, and through which we filter experience.

So we let loose, go easy on ourselves, and drop into the nowscape of being with the gentle but firm intention to be undistracted, utterly attentive, and without "making" anything. Second, and equally importantly, since the mind will be fabricating anyway, for all our intentions for it not to, we watch the fabricating tendency itself and inquire into what the watching capacity, the knowing capacity really is. The knowing capacity becomes intimate with the fabrications, not so much through thought but through feel. We recognize the proliferations and the endless construction projects of the mind, and how easily we get absorbed in them, how easily we get emotionally involved in them. We recognize how easily we cling to them and have opinions about them, whether positive or negative, pleasant or unpleasant. When it comes right down to it, all of this, we see, is mere fabrication: ideas and opinions, most of them highly conditioned, repetitive, confining, and even wrong. So we keep watching the mind's constructs arise and pass away. We rest in awareness itself, beyond thinking altogether, even thoughts of watching and knowing. We rest in this awareness momentarily, and this "momentarily" is itself beyond time.

Over time, such timeless moments emerge out of the background of endless proliferations and fabrications and are seen and known because they become more familiar to us and therefore more visible and more accessible. We are naturally drawn to reside in undisturbed peacefulness (equanimity) and clarity no matter what is happening. We have momentarily at least gotten out of our own way, at which point the way becomes evident, bright, and undisturbed, even when the proverbial stuff is hitting the proverbial fan, maybe even especially when the proverbial stuff is hitting the proverbial fan.

And if we do get caught up in fabrications in any particular moment, it might even occur to us to check the circuit breakers—the ones in the basement, and especially the ones in the mind.

Any Ideal of Practice Is Just Another Fabrication

Of course, what was just said in the last chapter is also just a view and thus, in some way, lends itself to idealization. It is all too easy to idealize the notion of mindfulness practice, or of our own practice, or fall into notions of attainment and, as we have seen, special states of mind, and then stay stuck in our concepts and ideals of practice for years without seeing that they are themselves fabrications, big ones.

For getting stuck over and over again is nothing other than practice too, as long as we are willing to see it and work with it through continually letting go, and through continual kindness toward ourselves. One thing is virtually certain. We will get stuck over and over again in the short run no matter what we do or think, because that is the nature of the unexamined and underdeveloped mind.

We will fabricate problems and everything else that the mind and its ongoing story of me can come up with or react to over and over again. And once we get into meditation, we will do it about meditation as much if not more than we do it about everything else in our lives. That is only natural, and it is not necessarily a problem! Like all fabrications and all proliferations of mind, it is simply part of the landscape of practice. The challenge, and it is a huge and unrelenting one, is to stay mindful even as we are getting stuck, or to recover mindfulness as quickly as we can after we lose our minds and succumb to our countless insecure, fear-driven, ingrained, and mindless habits.

This is not an ideal. But it is hard work. It requires an attitude that insists that there is no other time than now, no matter what is occurring, no matter how conflicted or in turmoil you may feel. There is simply no other, better occasion to be awake, no other, better moment, ever, in which to be aware. And so it is literally, as the song says, now or never. Choosing now, we open to it and rest in awareness itself. Now we can act—spontaneously—in the nowscape, out of that very dimension of being and knowing, in the simplest and purest of ways, embodying wholeness and wisdom, not through thinking or fabrication, but because wholeness and wisdom are what and who we already are—our H_2O, our true nature—but, sadly, in terms of our own potential, keep forgetting.

*

The Great Way is not difficult
for those not attached to preferences.
When love and hate are both absent
everything becomes clear and undisguised.

⋮

If you wish to move in the One Way
do not dislike even the world of senses and ideas.
Indeed, to accept them fully
is identical with Enlightenment…

SENG-TS'AN, third Zen Patriarch (circa 600 CE) "Verses on the Faith-Mind" (*Hsin-Hsin Ming*)

You Want to
Make Something of It?

When I was growing up in New York City—Washington Heights to be specific—these were fighting words. They got said a lot. Someone would make an insulting comment to someone else, and the insultee would say, "You want to make something of it?" (Actually it came out sounding more like *you wanna*...). And if the original guy said, "Yeah, I do wanna make something of it," then they would start pushing each other and maybe escalate to something more.

You want to make something of it? An interesting challenge, especially for rough-and-tumble street kids in the 1950s.

In light of what we have been saying about the mind and its tendencies to fabricate, it is interesting for me now to reflect on why, as adolescent boys, we would say such a thing. In the street argot of the day, to make something of it meant to pursue it further, take it to the next level. You were standing up for yourself, and forcing the insulting party to back down or back up what he was saying. But if *you*, the insultee, wanted to make something of it, that also meant that the challenge had become real for you, that it had gotten under your skin, that you were hooked and taking it personally, and that it was important to respond to the insinuation, however off-the-wall, if only out of adolescent ennui, and of course, to defend your "reputation" on the block.

Typically it was an outrageous sexually charged put-down directed at some member of the other guy's family, usually his mother, and it could work either way so either side could want to make something of it and say that to the other side. After a while it didn't even matter what the original offense was, or who started it. It was just: "You wanna make something of it?" "Yeah. I wanna make something of it if you wanna make something of it...."

But there was a socially acceptable way of letting it go. And if you went that route, you didn't lose face, either as the insulter or the insultee. If you were cool, relaxed, nonchalant, humor-full, in other words, equanimous and transparent to the insult, not taking it personally, especially if you were on the receiving end of it, you could just let it go (since it was totally stupid and bogus and nonsensical anyway, as was the whole interchange) and everything would be OK.

But if either one of you took the meaning seriously and let yourself get insulted, even though you both knew it was all in jest really, then—especially if you were on the receiving end—you would get angry, and you usually wanted to hurt the other person for saying such a thing about your mother or your sister, which was exactly what the other person wanted, just to bait you into losing your composure. It was all totally ridiculous, but what else was there to do hanging out on street corners in the late fifties and being bored in between stickball games or other street sports indigenous only to the city? (People tell me that such antics and rituals go on to this very day, although now such edgy energies are also expressed through hip-hop and rapping, which are much more creative, poetic, nuanced, and socially aware than anything we ever came up with.)

But wait just a minute! When you come right down to it, what *don't* we make something of? We make something out of virtually anything and everything. And in doing so, we get caught. Our adolescent street ritual was really all about playing around with attachment and non-attachment. If you got caught by the words and the thoughts, which were designed as juicy bait to really hook you, then you had to fight to preserve your "honor." But if you didn't take it to heart, if you didn't snap at the bait but let it go by, then there was no problem. Your so-called honor or self-esteem was never in any danger in the first place.

So this ritual we used to subject each other to endlessly actually reveals at its core an intimate intuitive understanding of the same teaching that Soen Sa Nim was emphasizing, namely, "You make, you have." The interchange was pure Zen, a form of what Soen Sa Nim called "Dharma combat."

I find all this pretty interesting to contemplate, especially since no one taught it to us as a mode of inquiry or self-understanding. It was homegrown in Washington Heights. It may not have taken us very far, but it was on to something way beyond our conscious understanding, and you could say, in its own way, wise.

You make problem, you have problem. You make insult, you have insult. You make an interpretation, you have an interpretation, you make fear, you have fear, you make anger, you have anger. There are infinite opportunities for us to get stuck in fabrication in our own mind, for us to latch on to some event or other and make it into something, something much more than it really is. This is the origin of a huge amount of grief and mania. If we make something of our perceptions, some big story, such as "they" don't love me, or "they" don't respect me, or "things are not supposed to have happened like this," or "my body is no good," or "my life is a failure," or "I'm the king of the world," the very model of a modern major general or movie star, or whatever it is for you, rather than seeing the essential emptiness/fullness of events and residing in our hearts with acceptance and equanimity, in the integrity of spacious, openhearted, choiceless awareness, we might be right, or we might be wrong, we might be requited, or we might not ever be, but we will never know peace, and we will never see the big picture, beyond the stories, big and little, we are telling ourselves and then forgetting that we made up, fabricated, all by ourselves.

Our "I" will always interfere with and veil our eyes, our ears, our nose, our tongue, our skin, our hearts and minds, and our moments.

In seeing our own fabrications arise moment by moment, maybe we can let them go without getting caught by them so much of the time. And maybe we might see it more rapidly when we are invariably caught by them. It's a worthy challenge, and a worthy practice.

So let me ask you now: "Do you want to make something of it?"

Watch out!

Who Won the Super Bowl?

One year, I was on a two-week silent meditation retreat that began the weekend of the 2002 Super Bowl. It was only the third time that the New England Patriots had made it there, and they had never won. The drama was increased for New England fans at the time because of the dismal record of the Boston Red Sox in the World Series, never having won since 1918, after trading Babe Ruth to the New York Yankees in 1919.*

Adding to the drama, the regular New England quarterback, Drew Bledsoe, their star player, had been seriously injured in the second game of the season and had been replaced by his until-then unknown second-year backup, Tom Brady. Brady wound up taking the team all the way to the playoffs, then getting injured in the game that determined the division championship and whether they would go to the Super Bowl. Bledsoe, who hadn't played since his injury several months earlier, stepped in and engineered with grace and ease a victory over the heavily favored Pittsburgh Steelers.

The fans bonded with both these men, who were endlessly fawned over in the local media and extolled for how kind, selfless, and gracious they were being about their predicament and the multiple

---

* Of course, they later went on to win the World Series twice under Terry Francona, in 2004 and 2007, and again in 2013, under John Farrell. The 2004 win broke "The Curse" that bedeviled Boston fans for almost a century.

ironies of it. New England was going to the Super Bowl. That we knew. The question was, who would wind up quarterbacking? And whoever it was, could the team possibly win against the heavily favored St. Louis Rams?

That is how I left it and the media frenzy when the retreat started Friday night. We were to be silent and sequestered from the outside world, except for possible emergencies, for from fourteen days to two months, depending on how long we had signed up for. During a talk Sunday evening, one of the teachers actually brought up the Super Bowl as an example of what we were renouncing by attending the retreat. He was teasing us a little in a good-natured way, but he did drop the comment that he would be willing to tell us the outcome of the game during individual interviews, if we really wanted to know. I made a mental note to remember to ask him.

But by the time my first interview with him came around the next morning, my attention was so taken up with the richness of experiencing the sitting and the walking practices that comprised the major time commitment of the retreat, it didn't even cross my mind to ask about the Super Bowl when I had the chance. This in spite of having inevitably gotten caught up in all the hoopla around it back in Boston just like many other people, whether they were die-hard Patriot fans or not. It amazed me, when I remembered about it later, that something I had had so much enthusiasm for had gone by the boards so fast. The thought occurred to me to ask him the next time I saw him, and then, on thinking about it, I decided not to. My seeing of it went this way:

What difference does it make to me now? Whoever won has already won, and I will find out soon enough. The game is over. Why do I need or want to know who won at this point? If New England won, my mind will just be full of thoughts about it, and if New England lost, my mind will be filled with a whole range of other thoughts about it. Either way, my elation if they won or my suffering if they lost will be purely vicarious, short-lived, and inconsequential. When you come right down to it, knowing the outcome has nothing to do with me or my life, even though I live in New England, even though I watched the game in which Bledsoe led the team to victory, even though I knew my children would be watching the game and would have gotten caught up in it, and would have been pleased if the Patriots had won. I came to see that wanting to know was itself an attachment to a certain kind of fiction, a way to fill my mind with another story I could get entangled in, a way of identifying with a particular outcome of an event that was really, at best, incidental to my life, and totally irrelevant to the work of the retreat. The work of the retreat, the whole reason I chose to be there, the whole reason I rearranged my life to be there even though it meant missing a lot of things, the least of which was the Super Bowl, was to be as awake as possible to present-moment experience in an admittedly and deliberately highly simplified and sequestered environment, one that is extremely hard to arrange, but which is structured precisely so that one can experience the luxury of not having external information that is not directly relevant to one's life intruding itself into the stream of unfolding experience, as it usually does so incessantly and with our unending, if often unconscious and sometimes highly addictive, collaboration.

Parenthetically, I am recounting all this in a way that suggests that my mind was utterly preoccupied with the Super Bowl, regardless of whether I found out who won or not. In fact, it all transpired in a few moments, some as thinking, some as pure seeing. It appeared, lingered, dissolved, and disappeared within a few minutes. The reconstructing of it here, in retrospect, takes a lot of words and thoughts to express.

I then saw the Super Bowl in an even bigger frame. For all the excitement of spectator sports and the real athletic skill and virtuosity it sometimes manifests, and the good feelings in the city stemming from its team's successes, I saw the huge colossus behind such an engineered event...the millions of dollars spent by the league and by the teams, the millions spent on advertising, the huge media hype that

builds over the season culminating in the extravagance of the inflat-
edly named "Super Bowl" and then, the hype after the game, the salary
bonanzas for key winners, and then the wait to repeat the whole thing
the next year. Some fans are elated because their team won, some fans
are depressed because their team lost, but the corporate-media feast is
the big winner every year. It never loses. That's the way the game is set
up, like house rules at a casino.

So that year, 2002—which was the only year for decades in which
I got fairly interested in pro football, even though I played football as
a boy, down on the grass near the Little Red Lighthouse, under the
looming George Washington Bridge, and loved the game, and loved
watching the early Super Bowls—because I was on retreat, I found
myself stepping away and settling into a richness that always lies right
under my nose, as close as this breath, any breath, whether I am on
retreat or not.

An aside: A year and a half earlier, I attended a retreat for about a
week during the 2000 presidential election. The morning after Election Day, the retreatants were given the option of lifting up a piece
of blank paper on the bulletin board that shielded the result from
sight, so that only those who really wanted to know would be able
to see who had been elected president. The rest could find out when
the retreat was over. That retreat went until mid-December. Under
the piece of paper, day after day, the message was always the same
inconceivable one: "We don't know yet." Imagine how confused the
meditators were who wanted to know and knew only that nobody did,
without any of the story of why! A perfect example of truth trumping
fiction, although now, almost two decades later, using this verb has an
entirely different range of dysphoric meanings.

I did ultimately find out who won the Super Bowl that year. It was
New England in a fairy-tale win. Brady led the team downfield in the
final eighty-one seconds of the game, with the score tied at 17–17 (the

Patriots led at one point 17–3), into field goal position, and the Patriot kicker, Adam Vinatieri, made it 20–17 in the final seconds. Soon afterward, Bledsoe was traded to Buffalo and was no longer a Patriot. Once again, an example of the law of impermanence at work. Hopefully Bledsoe had no attachments to New England. But of course he must have had some. Perhaps he dealt with them. And perhaps his Boston fans eventually dealt with their attachment to him. What else was there to do?

But during the retreat, since I had been unable to watch the game itself, examining whether I even wanted to know about it after the fact, although part of me certainly did, when my attention had already turned in another direction, presented its own interesting set of challenges and insights that left me feeling that whoever had won the Super Bowl, the game we were playing on the retreat, the game of being present for life itself, eclipsed all bowls, however super.

Reading the papers our kids saved for us a month later, I felt elated at the story of New England's good fortune and also felt how empty and contrived the whole thing was at the same time. It was a compelling event for some people at the time of its unfolding. Past that moment, it became just another sports story for the record books, a source of championship T-shirts, and reminiscences for a few die-hard fans. It came and it went. It arose, it passed away. It was, indeed, empty of any enduring reality. It was also fun, and just what it was, no more, no less.

Postscript: Two years later, in 2004, Tom Brady's Patriots won the Super Bowl again—against the Carolina Panthers, and again, they won it in the final seconds with a Vinatieri field goal. This time I was leading a mindfulness retreat for the heads of the clinical departments at Duke Medical School that started that evening. Because it was North Carolina, we "had" to watch the game. So I proposed that we build watching it into the retreat itself, as a form of mindfulness practice—namely, that we try to watch it mindfully, to be aware of the effects it was having on us and what we were bringing to it, especially in terms of attachment to the outcome. Unfortunately, I didn't have the presence of mind to suggest at the beginning that we watch it with the sound off, so we could better take it in, and hear our own inner commentary. I wish I had.

*

In a sense, you could say that mindfulness is really the only game in town, the only game that we ordinary folks get to play in if we want to, whether we watch Super Bowls or not, whether we are sports enthusiasts or not, whether we are athletes or not. With mindfulness, just playing is winning—because you are alive now...and...you know it.

*

Second postscript: Fifteen years later, in 2018 Tom Brady is still playing, at age 40, having won four Super Bowls. He is considered one of the greatest quarterbacks ever, if not the greatest, although the Patriots, to the huge disappointment of New England fans, inconceivably lost in the Super Bowl in 2017 to the upstart Philadelphia Eagles.

Now we know for certain some of the hidden costs of the game, denied for decades by the NFL. I am speaking about chronic traumatic encephalopathy, CTE, the concussive effects on the brain experienced by so many players in the NFL and the unending downstream suffering, loss, and grief they and their families live with as a result. Famed Patriot linebacker, Junior Seau committed suicide at age 43. Patriot Aaron Hernandez was found guilty of murder and committed suicide in prison at age 27. His brain was found to be severely damaged by CTE, as has been the case for so many other NFL players. Yet in 2017, the president of the United States complained that the game is not violent enough, and that penalties for hits to the head are "ruining the game." He also condemned players who do not stand for the playing of the national anthem, calling the protesters "sons of bitches." One player opined: "I guess we are all sons of bitches now."

In 2016, Colin Kaepernick, former quarterback for the San Francisco 49ers had started a trend by taking a knee during the playing of the national anthem, in sympathy with the victims of police brutality and murder in the African American community. It was taken up by entire teams for a time in 2017 in the wake of Trump's invective, and many prominent players in the NBA (National Basketball Association) expressed strong political statements in solidarity with those athletes supporting greater social justice for people of color. Kaepernick gave away one million dollars in 2016 in support of groups working in oppressed inner-city communities and sponsors an annual "know your rights" camp to "raise awareness on higher education, self-empowerment, and instruction to properly interact with law enforcement in various scenarios" for young people of color.

So, hardly surprising, the universe of American football continues to mirror the society that gave rise to it. Who wins the Super Bowl each year pales in comparison to what is really unfolding, whether you love the game or not. How might we hold that in awareness? How might we hold in awareness whatever we are a devoted fan of that might have a toxic shadow side?*

---

* For a brilliant treatment of this very human behavior to take sides in sporting events and its relationship to tribalism, evolutionary biology, politics, and the "emptiness" of inherent existence (See Book 1, "Emptiness"), see Robert Wright, *Why Buddhism Is True*, Simon & Schuster, New York, 2017: 181–185.

Arrogance and Entitlement

Because we can at times have the experience of being able to control things for a moment or two in our lives, there is a subtle way in which we can fall into telling ourselves stories about the way things are supposed to work out more generally. Planes are supposed to leave and arrive on time. My flight, underscore the "my," is not supposed to be canceled because I have got to get where I am supposed to be by a particular time for such and such a reason. (Can you feel the indignation, the self-centeredness, and the self-importance rising up?) People are supposed to be reliable and do what they said they would, especially when dealing with me. Investments are supposed to increase in value. Children are supposed to be safe. Our bodies are supposed to stay healthy if we eat right and exercise regularly.

The more things go "our way" for a while, the more we can convince ourselves that that is the way it is supposed to be. And when things don't go "our way," which sooner or later they will not, we can get angry, disappointed, depressed, devastated, forgetting that it was never "supposed to be" any one way at all. How our lives unfold is virtually never exactly the way we think they will, or plan for them to, or desire that they do. It is never entirely under our control. Yet we persist in thinking that things should be a certain way, that I should not have to suffer this indignity, or that loss, or should be treated this way and certainly not that way; and that the world should be a certain way, that wars shouldn't happen, or earthquakes. And the more powerful we are in terms of our status in an organization or within society, or even within the society of our own head (recall the saying that "he was a legend in his own mind"), the more susceptible we become to intimations of our own infallibility, to an arrogance that forgets that all things change in ways that are uncertain, that nothing is fixed for long, and that we are all subject to the law of impermanence. Such a simple, elegant realization. It could readily, if kept in mind, counterbalance our natural tendencies toward arrogance and self-importance, and help us to learn how to live more in line with the dharma, the tao, with the lawfulness of all things, especially in the face of hardships, of dukkha, of anguish—if only we would take it to heart.

Whatever the particulars—and it is the particulars that are always the hardest to accept because, in general, we do know that things unfold in ways that only have some vague correspondence to our fantasies and fears—upon deeper scrutiny, it always turns out that it was merely a story we wound up telling ourselves, perhaps unconsciously, and that story, those unexamined images and that stream of feelings, wound up seducing us into a pervasive unawareness and at taking things for granted just when we most needed to keep our wits about us. For we seem to be perpetually at risk of being seduced by the appearance of things, by the spells of *samsara* and *maya*, Sanskrit terms for the illusory play of the sensory world, so often not entirely perceived and comprehended with any clarity, and by which we are so easily enticed into a trance of delusion and illusion, including barely conscious intimations of immortality or omnipotence or privilege on the part of our "small" self.

No doubt about it. Luck and hard work *can* come together, and often do, especially in a stable society of multiple opportunities and mostly benevolent, if imperfect, laws that honor the life and freedom of the individual at least in principle* as well as the rights of

---

* Although, for a compelling critical perspective on the professed ideal of democracy versus the actuality, see Chomsky, N. *Who Rules the World?* Henry Holt, New York, 2016; and Zinn, H. *A People's History of the United States*, HarperCollins, New York, 1980, 2003.

communities of people, to create a semblance of balance, stability, and "progress" in our personal life or our professional life, or, if we are really lucky, in both. Things are much less that way, much more overtly chaotic in many so-called developing countries. But in so-called developed countries, things can have the appearance of going "according to plan" for a long time, especially during periods of what passes for "peacetime." But subtle feelings of satisfaction at having things turn out "right" over and over again can work a deception on us if they gradually turn into feelings of "self"-satisfaction, even entitlement, because things have unfolded the way we thought they should up to now. Then we are vulnerable to rude awakenings, when the situation changes in ways that are not in accord with our scenario, with our maps of how things are in this world, when we are caught napping.

When all of a sudden we find that things are not as we thought, hoped, expected, required, counted on, blindly believed, whether on the personal level, the professional level, the societal level, or the global level, it is indeed a big wake-up call, perhaps a very rude and painful awakening. We discover that things were not always the way we thought they were, and may not have been that way all along. Perhaps they never were. They may have just appeared that way for a time. We may have been deluded from the start—a masquerade we might have been all too happy to participate in. This self-deception can happen in individuals or in society more broadly. It can happen in families. It can also happen for countries. It is very easy to lose one's way, especially if we collaborate in the delusion.

Inevitably, if our trajectory on this planet is not foreshortened, whether we like it or not, whether we ever come to terms with it or not, we grow old, often in ways that weren't part of our scenario for how it was supposed to happen for us. We can gradually but inexorably lose our minds to Alzheimer's disease or our body to other egregious or more subtle afflictions. We may lose people we love in ways we never imagined. We die deaths not consistent with our imaginings.

The stock market goes down after years of going up for reasons that were not entirely healthy, but what the hell, where else can you make money like this? Corporate greed, rogue accounting practices, and unethical behavior are revealed as endemic in companies that spend billions annually to create images of their own impeccability and infallibility, and we are somehow shocked. All the same, the next day or the next year, it is all pretty much forgotten. Until it repeats.

Wake-up calls just highlight our chronic somnambulance. We are caught believing in and living in a dream reality, invested in it emotionally, unwilling and unable to see through it because of our own personal attachment to the dream, especially if it seems a good one, and lots of people seem to share in it. A certain subtle or perhaps not-so-subtle arrogance may have crept into our hearts, through our own internal life requirement that things be as we want them to be, worked for them to be, thought them to be, and dreamed that they were. A thin mist of entitlement may have crept in, blanketing everything in the belief that things should pretty much always work out for me and mine, as planned, as hoped for. Now, in a moment of revelation, events change and we see that it is "not always so" in the words of the late Zen Master Shunryu Suzuki. We see how we may have been blinded to our own attachment to certainty, and to the comfort and perhaps social or racial privilege of having had things go "our way" for long stretches of time, or lived in the illusion of it even as it wasn't so. Or perhaps we forgot that "our way" is not necessarily what we think our way is. Maybe we need to be asking, "What is my way with a capital W?" Maybe our societies, our countries, and the world need to be asking a similar question.

Once rudely awakened, or awakened by any other path, the real challenge is not to fall back asleep and spin off into perpetual resentment and blaming and the nightmares they proliferate into. For the sleep habit, the allure of *samsara*, is a strong one and requires a strong commitment to wakefulness to counteract.

There is no blame here, or put differently, plenty of blame to go around. It is inevitable that we will get caught in our own dreams, especially when the entire society conspires to show only one side of its face to itself, the other side denied, in shadow. But rather than getting caught in blaming we can also wake up from these dreams to something larger and truer, and therefore, ultimately, more healing if also more painful. To wake up, we need to give up a clinging we may have been barely aware of into a larger view, truer, more sobering, but also more real and therefore liberating and transformative. A place we can reside in and from which we can meet the world in an entirely adequate way, now, either without delusions—which may be nigh impossible for us, when you throw in the subtle ones—or at the very least aware of them fairly quickly when they do creep in.

That something larger, that larger view must needs include a fundamental recognition of the increase in human anguish when anything at all is clung to to enhance self-satisfaction or power or privilege as opposed to cared for to enhance the well-being of others.

That something larger includes recognizing that things that we desire to stay the same and that we cling to will inevitably change and the things that we so much want to change will seem to hold still and resist change the more we try to force them to move as we wish. And it includes recognizing that the "laws" that are driving these events are fundamentally impersonal, having to do with causes and conditions that are often influenced by our own individual and collective greed, hatred, ignorance, and our complacent delusion and collusion. And it includes recognizing that these ever-changing causes and conditions drive our reactive phase changes while obscuring our essential nature that is bigger than and more fundamental than any or all of the sleep states we fall into.

We do not have to go back to sleep, if we manage to wake up at all. But without maintaining some kind of mindfulness practice as a love affair with what is most important and necessary to keep in mind and embody, it is highly likely that when the conditions are right, we will be seduced into another nice dream, and forget again. Practicing staying awake, we have more of a chance to perceive our myopia and take steps to correct it. We can smell not just the roses, but the odor of our own arrogance and entitlement wafting back in, however subtle. In doing so, we can come relatively quickly to our senses and rest in how things actually are. We can trust in our own presence of mind and heart when mind and heart no longer need to tell themselves anything but instead can simply be available, remain wide open in awareness, and act fearlessly and lovingly without expectation out of that awareness, in the face of things as they actually are right now.

*

. . . you know the sprout is hidden inside the seed.
We are all struggling; none of us has gone far.
Let your arrogance go, and look around inside.

The blue sky opens out farther and farther,
the daily sense of failure goes away,
the damage I have done to myself fades,
a million suns come forward with light,
when I sit firmly in that world.

KABIR
Translated by Robert Bly

Death

Since impermanence, emptiness, and selflessness have been such underlying themes in our explorations, consider once again for a moment the fleetingness of life. Our bodies, quantized condensations of vital protoplasm—certainly among the most complex and differentiated conglomerations of matter and energy we know of in the universe—arise and pass away. And with their passing fade and pass the details of each individual life and its personal expression. What is left are the photographs, the home videos, whatever migrated to YouTube or Facebook, the memories, the little triumphs and gestures, the stories we who are still here recall or tell ourselves silently about who someone was or wasn't; and about the missed moments too: what might have happened but didn't, what could have been but wasn't.

Yet life itself, the living, pulsating interconnected web to which all organisms belong, goes on. In a very real sense, bodies are just a way for the genes to pass themselves along in various combinations that ensure their survival under changing circumstances. We *think* we are in charge, but our genes have a life of their own. And while we have a relatively brief life, theirs is immeasurably longer. We organisms could be seen as merely a by-product of their romping about in the world. Richard Dawkins's poignant term for this perspective is the "selfish" gene. Talk about emptiness!

O dark dark dark. They all go into the dark,
The vacant interstellar spaces, the vacant into the vacant,
The captains, merchants, bankers, eminent men of letters,
The generous patrons of art, the statesmen and the rulers,
Distinguished civil servants, chairmen of many committees,
Industrial lords and petty contractors, all go into the dark...

And we all go with them...

T. S. ELIOT, "East Coker," *Four Quartets*

Now all my teachers are dead except silence.

W. S. MERWIN

All the prominent scientists of an earlier generation who contributed to shaping molecular biology when I was a graduate student, even though they tended to work long into their seventies and eighties, are at this point soon to retire, long retired, or dead. Their legacy endures, often increasingly anonymously. Their hard-won knowledge gained over a lifetime's career fed younger generations of scientists and science itself, and provided the platform for what is unfolding in laboratories now. My teachers would have marveled at the speed at which new understandings are emerging, at the level of automation in the manipulation of genes and organisms routinely going on every day in labs around the world, and at the speed with which data and papers are shared. And they might have cringed and swallowed hard, I would guess, at the ethical dilemmas inherent in being so close to being able to shape life in ways that were never possible before, by human minds that are unbelievably and admirably precocious in some ways, yet morally, even emotionally, underdeveloped, sometimes infantile, ignorant, or even dangerous in so many others.

I have seen scientists metaphorically salivating at the possibility of life extension, if not virtual immortality, through isolating and manipulating what are called senescence genes, those stretches of DNA in the genome that seem to influence the longevity of species. Some describe aging as a potentially curable disease.

We all have moments, I suppose, when we long for immortality, to keep going forever. But in what form? At what age? At what cost to ourselves, to others, and to the planet? We have never before had to face such prospects, and our track record so far suggests we are ill equipped for doing so. But we may be faced with having to plumb the depths of the mind's capacity for wisdom rather quickly or collectively suffer consequences of undreamed of, potentially Promethean, proportions.

Some time ago, biologists won the Nobel Prize for elucidating the mechanism of apoptosis—programmed cell death. For unbeknownst to many of us, death is actually genetically programmed into life. Many of our perfectly healthy cells actually need to die for the overall organism to grow and optimize itself. This selective cell death occurs as our limbs and organ systems are developing in utero, and this dying of certain cells continues throughout our lives. In fact, it is absolutely necessary for our lives that many of our cells will die, and know when to do it. A compelling biological example of nonattachment to a small sense of self.

Immortality in cells is cancer. Cancer cells don't get the message that this growing and dividing needs to be in the service of the larger whole, and therefore modulated, regulated as needed, kept under flexible control. In fact, at different rates, all of our cells live for a time and then die, to be replaced by new cells. This is true for our skin and the lining of our stomach and intestines, for muscle and nerve cells, for blood cells, for bone cells.

There is both a coming into form and going out of form. Without the going, there can be no coming, or becoming. Maybe even our cells are trying to tell us that death is not such a bad thing, and nothing to be feared. Maybe our knowing of death, our ability to foretell its inevitability yet not know the timing of it is a goad for us to wake up to our lives, to live them while we can, fully, passionately, wisely, lovingly, joyfully, and without attachment.

For we are dying a little every day, just as we are being born a little every day. We die with each out-breath, only to be breathed back to life with the next in-breath. We have been dying from the beginning. That dying is perpetually cleaning out our house and making room for something new. And so, if we are aware of this dynamical process that is intrinsic to life expressing itself in the form of individual bodies, and if we align ourselves with this understanding in our own hearts, we can continue growing into ourselves while we have the chance, into what is most meaningful to us, building on what we already are, starting with where we already are, knowing that this is it. And in the larger perspective of wholeness, knowing that it never gets any better than this because all is always now. Recall those lines of Kabir:

Friend, hope for the guest while you are alive.
Jump into experience while you are alive
Think... and think... while you are alive.
What you call "salvation" belongs to the time before death.

If you don't break your ropes while you're alive,
do you think
ghosts will do it after?

The idea that the soul will join with the ecstatic
just because the body is rotten—
that is all fantasy.
What is found now is found then.
If you find nothing now,
you will simply end up with an apartment in the City of Death.

If you make love with the divine now, in the next life
you will have the face of satisfied desire...

KABIR
Translated by Robert Bly

*

And from Albert Einstein:

With the departure from this strange world, he now has gone a little ahead of me. This is of no significance. For us believing physicists, the separation between past, present, and future has only the meaning of an illusion, albeit a tenacious one.

ALBERT EINSTEIN,
upon hearing of the death of his close friend,
Michelangelo Besso

DYING BEFORE YOU DIE

When I was writing my Ph.D. thesis, I wanted to give at least a nod to the existential struggle it had been for me, and to my discovery of meditation and yoga and how liberating and life-saving they had been. So I put, on a page by itself right after the title page, the cryptic phrase:

"He who dies before he dies does not die when he dies."

I don't even remember where I got it.

My defense committee consisted of six men and one woman, all in their late-forties to late-fifties, all remarkably creative and successful. They were luminaries at the cutting edges of molecular biology, in a department that was always ranked at the very top of annual national rating schemes. Most were members of the prestigious National Academy of Sciences, including my thesis advisor, Salvador Luria, who had shared the Nobel Prize in medicine and physiology in 1969 for his highly imaginative statistical demonstration, done decades earlier in collaboration with the physicist Max Delbruck, that mutations in bacteria occur spontaneously and randomly. Luria's most famous graduate student was Jim Watson, the co-discoverer, along with Francis Crick, of the double helical structure of DNA, who won the Nobel Prize for that seminal discovery seven years before Luria won his.*

What amazed me was that the first part of my thesis defense that day centered not around the content of the thesis and the experimental work I had done but on that opening aphorism. Someone started off with a question about it, maybe just to put me at my ease before diving into the defense proper. But one question led to another, and their questions displayed genuine curiosity. They clearly wanted to know what dying *before* you die meant and why I had put it in my thesis. At their urging, I explained that to me, it was referring to the death of one's attachment to a narrow view of life centered on one's own ego, that self-preoccupied, self-constructed story-lens of at best dubious accuracy through which we see everything within the inflated context of our own self-cherishing habit that features us, although we would be reluctant to admit it, as the undisputed center of the universe.

Dying before you die meant waking up to a larger reality beyond the narrowly constrained view one gets through one's own ego and self-centered preoccupations—a reality that is not knowable merely through one's limited ideas and opinions and highly conditioned preferences and aversions, especially those that remain unexamined. It meant becoming conscious, not in the sense of intellectually knowledgeable but more in the sense of directly *feeling and keeping in mind* the fleeting nature of life and of all our relationships, and of life's ultimately impersonal nature. Within such a coordinate system, one could then choose purposefully, to whatever degree one could manage it, to live outside the routinized automaticity that frequently seduces

---

* Although part of the backstory is that the X-ray crystallographic data Watson and Crick used in their discovery was obtained from Rosalind Franklin, a colleague who died of cancer at age 37, but who was not credited until long after her death with providing the critical data to support the double helix structure. Had she lived longer, in all likelihood, she might have won a Nobel Prize in Chemistry along with her student and collaborator, Aron Klug, who did receive that recognition in 1982.

us through small-minded ambitions and fears and thereby numbs us to
the beauty and the mystery of life (even as biologists) and prevents us
from looking more creatively into the deep nature of things, including ourselves (even as scientists) as living organisms with unknown
and fleeting lifespans, behind all the surface appearances and the stories we tell ourselves about who we are.

Of course, I can't remember verbatim what I said, but the gist
went something like that.

As for not dying when you die, I continued, to me it meant that if
you lead a wakeful life while you are alive, and observe the continually
self-constructing ego energy without getting caught up in it, there comes
a realization that this overwhelmingly dominant self-referencing habit
is an inaccurate and fundamentally empty construct, and that strictly
speaking, there is no you to die. What dies when you die before death is
the concept of a special, concrete, isolated "I." Once you realize that, there
is no death at any time except as a thought in the mind, and no one to die
either. That is why the Buddha spoke of liberation as "the Deathless."

I am sure that at age twenty-seven I responded to their questioning with great sincerity but also, in hindsight, with perhaps a seriousness and self-assurance at least skirting the edges of, if not falling
full-bore into, the arrogant. I was certainly at high risk, under the circumstances, of falling into attachment to the view I was expounding
with such conviction. I had touched something, discovered something
through experimenting of a different kind, way outside the boundaries of their labs and their consensus reality (or at least, so I thought),
and of course, beyond the scope of our purpose for being assembled
on that day. I had somehow stumbled upon meditation and yoga during my time at MIT, and had developed a passion for what these dis-
ciplines had led to and revealed as possible. Nor did it feel to me that
these lenses for investigating reality were describing a realm entirely
beyond the boundaries of science. Far from it. But meditation and
yoga were clearly more than a little off the beaten path of molecular
biology and the subject of my thesis research. It is only in the past

twenty years or so that the serious scientific study of mindfulness meditation and related meditative practices has really taken off.

So once the subject of that opening quotation came up during my thesis defense, I guess I was hoping somewhere deep down in my heart to explain it to my mentors in a way they could understand, in spite of the unusual setting. Perhaps that was an unconscious, factor in putting the aphorism right up front in the thesis, although most of it had to do with a very conscious feeling that completing this life passage of my doctoral training was itself a death and a rebirth. The quotation was there to remind me of all of the travails and tribulations associated with that work and that time; and that I didn't have to cling to what it had been, that I could die to it.

Just having a philosophical conversation of this kind in the context of a thesis defense in the Biology Department at MIT was highly unusual. That the men in particular, who did most of the talking, were interested in that epigraph at all and wanted to talk about it was astonishing in that they were, as far as I knew, and I knew all of them fairly well, first and foremost supreme rationalists. I attributed their interest to the fact that they were at an age when they had probably already done the lion's share of what they were going to contribute to the world through their scientific work, and that they were becoming more aware of their own aging and mortality. Somehow, this mysterious poetic phrase about dying before you die, and the fact that it was being offered at the front of a piece of work by a student they all knew very well piqued their interest, and perhaps their egos. I am guessing that they must have already decided that the thesis work was good enough to pass, as long as I could talk intelligently about it in detail, so they were maybe a little more relaxed than they might have been if the circumstances had been otherwise, about taking time to talk about something so extraneous to the matter at hand. I am also guessing that the only woman in the room, Professor Annamaria Torriani-Gorini, was more than a little amused.

I don't recall the full extent of our conversation. No doubt there was a sense of amused tolerance, perhaps some politely raised eyebrows at my responses, but it was their ongoing questioning that prolonged our discussion, so it was clear to me that they actually wanted to talk about dying before you die. After a while, we launched into the defense proper.

That was in 1971. Almost fifty years later, Salva Luria is long gone, and I am older now by far than any of them were at the time. There was deep affection between Salva and me, but our relationship had a severe father/rebellious son, tempestuous quality to it, dosed heavily with his disapproval and perplexity at the life paths I was taking. The truth was, I drove him nuts a good deal of the time, and for perfectly understandable reasons, given who he was and who I was. But years later, he generously read a draft of *Full Catastrophe Living* in manuscript (I had asked him to critique it and give me his advice on how to improve it, as a way of reaching out to him) and ultimately, after he developed cancer, he asked me if I wouldn't come by and teach him a bit how to meditate. We had a few sessions together at his home (by that time, we actually lived a few blocks away from each other) in the year before he died, but as far as I know, it was not something that he really warmed to or intuitively grasped. So I would just stop by for a time on my way home from work to talk with him and see how he was doing. By that time, there was only sweetness between us

It only took decades for me to see that perhaps I was mostly espousing concepts at the time of the thesis defense, even though what I was saying was grounded in practice and in my nascent experience and understanding. They were nice concepts, good concepts, helpful concepts, concepts that helped me practice and also to endure particular kinds of existential rending that occurred during that time, but they were concepts all the same. This dying before you die proved more challenging than I had thought, and perhaps way deeper than I had tasted.

And of course, that is true even now. Guess what? As you move toward the horizon, you find that it is always receding. It is not a place that can be arrived at. There always seems to be some aspect of self that clings tenaciously to its own little story of I, me, and mine. A meditation practice is no guarantee of immunity from attachment or, for that matter, from delusion. All too easily, one merely shifts the clinging habit over to another class of concepts and fantasies. So-called spiritual communities are at particularly high risk for this very thing, the self-satisfied belief that your style of practice is the best practice, your view of the path the wisest view, your tradition and teachers the best tradition and teachers, and on it goes. Even as an individual, never mind a community, that is an easy trap to fall into and a hard one to extricate oneself from.

The challenge as I see it now is to sense the arising of any such story, however subtle, whatever its content, secular or sacred, and as part of our practice, to recognize it for what it is, another fabrication of the mind. Either we avoid becoming entangled in it, or we catch it quickly and gracefully whenever we do get entangled, and have a good laugh over it. In resting in awareness, the dying has already happened in this moment, and the knowing of such a moment fully met goes beyond concepts and words, however meaningful, however useful. Knowing this, words and concepts become powerful, because you know how to use them, and where they leave off.

*

*And so long as you haven't experienced
this: to die and so to grow,
you are only a troubled guest
on the dark earth.*

GOETHE, "The Holy Longing"

Dying Before You Die—Deux

By the time of my thesis defense, I had been practicing meditation in the Zen tradition for about five years. My first live exposure, ironically enough, also came at MIT, in 1966. Walking down one of the interminable two-tone green corridors one day, feeling rather alienated and out of sorts, in part because of the to-my-mind cynical and obscene war I felt we were perpetrating in Vietnam, my eye caught a flyer on one of the massive bulletin boards lining the hallways. It read, oddly: "The Three Pillars of Zen."

It was advertising a talk by Philip Kapleau, who had been a reporter at the Nuremberg War Crimes Tribunal and had then gone off to Japan for a number of years to practice Zen. He had been invited to MIT by Huston Smith, who was at the time a professor of philosophy and religion there. I had no idea what Zen was, or who Kapleau was, or Huston Smith for that matter, but for some reason, I went to the talk, which was held in the late afternoon, seminar hour.

What struck me right off was how few people showed up for it, not more than five or six out of the whole academic community of thousands. I no longer remember exactly what Kapleau said, except that he remarked in passing that when he started sitting in Japan, it was freezing cold in the monastery and there was no central heating. The conditions were Spartan and primitive. Yet his chronic stomach ulcers went away and never returned. Whatever else Kapleau said, it was my first time hearing somebody speak compellingly and from firsthand experience about meditation and about dharma. I remember feeling as I left the talk that I had stumbled onto something extremely important that couldn't have been more relevant to my life at the time, and to my sanity. So I started sitting on my own. Kapleau returned some time later and led a retreat over a weekend that helped deepen both my practice and my enthusiasm. Later, when his book *The Three Pillars of Zen* came out, I devoured it from cover to cover and kept going back to it for guidance with my nascent sitting practice.

That whole time as a graduate student felt like a death of sorts, and also a finding of new life. It signaled a gradual revealing of a new dimension to the original yearning that led me into science and biology in the first place, namely the impulse to investigate and understand the nature of life, the fact of consciousness itself, and the nature of reality—not just in the abstract, but as it manifested in my own life, my own mind, and my own life choices. The urge to follow the path of laboratory science was slowly dying, even though I remained as excited as ever about the discoveries that science makes possible. In parallel, the urge to understand myself through paying attention to the multiple dimensions of life and of being was becoming stronger and stronger. I was beginning to see life itself as the most interesting laboratory.

I was impressed during that time by the story of Ramana Maharshi, one of the great sages of the twentieth century who, one day, as a seventeen-year-old high school student with no previous spiritual training or interest, was overcome by an intense anxiety about death. He decided to go with what he was experiencing in the moment rather than resist, and to investigate it directly by asking, "What is dying?" He lay down and pretended to die, even holding his breath and imitating being overcome by rigor mortis.

What happened next was astonishing. According to his account, his personality permanently died then and there, on the spot. Apparently what was left was awareness itself, what he called the Self (with a capital *S*), an expression of identity with *Brahman*, or universal Self in his vocabulary. From that moment on, he taught the path of self-inquiry, the path of meditating on "Who am I?" People came to his modest hermitage at Tiruvannamalai, in Southern India, from all over the world to be in his presence, which was invariably described as emanating pure love, pure awareness, and a razor-sharp, mirror-like mind, empty of self, with which he responded in dialogue to all inquiries, however naïve, however profound. His serene smile looks out at me from a photograph across from my desk.

I've always associated Ramana's story with the corpse pose in yoga. Just intentionally assuming the corpse pose, on our backs, with our feet falling away from each other and our arms alongside the body but not touching it, the palms open to the ceiling or sky, affords ongoing opportunities to practice dying before we die. Lying stretched out in this way, utterly still except for the breath flowing as it will, we let the whole world be just as it is, unfold just as it is unfolding, as if, having died, it is simply going on in its way, but without us. All attachments sundered, already dead, so that there is nothing to cling to any further, we see, feel, and know that clinging itself is futile and our fears ultimately irrelevant. All we know is now, and that is spectacularly sufficient. If you are so inclined, you can inquire: "Who died?" "Who is doing yoga?" "Who is meditating?" "Who is breathing?" Even "Who is reading these words now?"

Dying to the past, dying to the future, dying to "I," "me," and "mine," we sense—lying in the corpse pose, as a corpse—the knowing quality or essence of mind, pure awareness, intrinsically empty of any self-concept, of all concept, of all thought, only that impersonal potential within which all thought and emotion arises. That sensing, that knowing is vibrantly alive here and, in the timelessness of this moment of now, forever—for you and for me.

So today, each moment in which we are alive, might be, actually is, a perfect day to die in this way, and so wake up.

Are you ready?

"Why wait any longer for the world to begin?"

Don't Know Mind

Soen Sa Nim used to sometimes act out for us how to practice with the koan, "What am I?" He would sit up straight, get a puzzled, quizzical look on his face, sit in silence for a few moments with his eyes closed, and then say, out loud, quite forcefully, "What am I?" He would string all the syllables together so it would come out, "Whatamiiiiiiii?" There would be silence for a moment and then, still with eyes closed and head tilted slightly, a puzzled expression on his face, out would come, again very forcefully, "Don't know!" It came out more like "Donnnnno!"

Whatamiiiiii?

Donnnno!

Then he would linger in the silence, in what he called "Don't know mind," just sitting there.

He was suggesting that it might not be a bad idea for us to practice like that, inwardly, in silence from time to time, at first with the words, but then way beyond the words. It was the questioning itself, the inquiry into the self, and the passion behind where the question was even coming from that were important. And the feeling, in the end, when it came right down to it, after all the investigating, after all the "not this, not this," underneath the thinking and all the vagaries of name and form, the feeling of simply not knowing, and resting in that not knowing, in all its poignancy, with full acceptance and spaciousness.

He would tell us to "keep don't know mind" in everything we did. "Only don't know!" he would bellow, and so a lot of his students would go around saying, "Only don't know" all the time, no matter what you asked them or said to them. It was hysterical. It was insufferable. It was also great training.

One day, Soen Sa Nim was being interviewed on a New York City radio station. At the end of the program, the host, the late Lex Hixon, a well-known Buddhist scholar and author, said to him: "Soen Sa Nim. Thank you for being on the show. I love your teachings and it has been a fascinating hour. But one thing I just don't get, and it has been puzzling me a lot as we have been talking. What is this donut mind you keep talking about? I just don't get it."

Soen Sa Nim roared with laughter. "Yes. That is it. 'Donut mind!' Nothing in the middle. Just air."

Arriving At Your Own Door

The time will come
when with elation,
you will greet yourself arriving
at your own door, in your own mirror,
and each will smile at the other's welcome,

and say sit here. Eat.
You will love again the stranger who was your self.
Give wine. Give bread. Give back your heart
to itself, to the stranger who has loved you

all your life, whom you ignored
for another, who knows you by heart.
Take down the love letters from the bookshelf,

the photographs, the desperate notes,
peel your own image from the mirror.
Sit. Feast on your life.

DEREK WALCOTT, "Love after Love"

By now, in our journey together up to this point, it shouldn't be that hard to recognize that in every moment, we are arriving at our own door. In any and every moment we could open it. In any and every moment, we might love again the stranger who was ourself, who knows us, as the poem says, by heart.

Ironically, we already know ourselves "by heart" in every sense of those two words, but we may have forgotten that we do. Arriving at our own door is all in the remembering, the re-membering, the reclaiming of that which we already are and belong to and have for too long ignored, having been carried seemingly farther and farther from home, yet at the same time, never being farther away than this breath and this moment. Can we wake up? Can we come to our senses? Can we be the knowing, that our awareness already is, and at the same time keep don't know mind and honor the not-knowing? Are they even different?

The time will come, the poet affirms. Yes, the time will come, but do we want it to be on our deathbeds when we wake up to who and what we actually are, as Thoreau foresaw could so easily happen when he said (see Book 1, "Introduction, page xxxiii" for the entire quote) "...and not, when I came to die, discover that I had not lived?" Or can that time be *this* time, be right now, where we are, as we are?

The time will come, yes, but only if we give ourselves over to waking up moment by moment, to coming to our senses moment by moment, and befriending and transcending our own underdeveloped minds. Only if we can perceive the chains of our robotic conditioning, especially our emotional conditioning and our view of who we think we are—peel our own image from the mirror—and in the perceiving, in seeing what is here to be seen, hearing what is here to be heard, watch the chains dissolve *in* the seeing, *in* the hearing, as we rotate back into our larger original beauty, as we greet ourself arriving at our own door, as we love again the stranger who was ourself. We can. We can. We will. We will. For what else, ultimately, is there for us to do?

How else, ultimately, are we to be free?

How else, ultimately, can we be who we already are?

How else are we to heal? How else are we to come to terms with things as they are?

And when, oh when, oh when is the moment this will happen?

"The time will come…" the poet says. Perhaps it already has. Only…Donnnno!

Perhaps it is time to practice, to feast on your life—as it is—right now, and now, and now, and now…

Acknowledgments

Since the origins of these four volumes go back a long way, there are a number of people to whom I wish to express my gratitude and indebtedness for their many contributions at various stages of the writing and publishing of these books.

For the initial volume, published in 2005, I would like to thank my dharma brother, Larry Rosenberg of the Cambridge Insight Meditation Center, as well as Larry Horwitz, and my father-in-law, the late Howard Zinn, for reading the entire manuscript back in the day and sharing their keen and creative insights with me. My thanks as well to Alan Wallace, Arthur Zajonc, Doug Tanner, and Richard Davidson and to Will Kabat-Zinn and Myla Kabat-Zinn for reading portions of the manuscript and giving me their wise council and feedback. I also thank the original publisher, Bob Miller, and the original editor, Will Schwalbe, now both at Flatiron Books, for their support and friendship, then and now.

Deep and special appreciation, gratitude, and indebtedness to my editor of the first volume, Michelle Howry, executive editor at Hachette Books, who helped midwife the form of the entire series; to Lauren Hummel for her key contributions to making sure all went well, and skillfully keeping all of the moving parts of this project on track; and to the entire Hachette team that worked so cooperatively and effectively on this series. Also, deep appreciation to Mauro DiPreta, vice president and publisher of Hachette Books, who stepped in to shepherd the last three volumes through the publication process when Michelle moved on.

While I have received support, encouragement, and advice from many, of course any inaccuracies or shortcomings in the text are entirely my own.

I wish to express enduring gratitude and respect to all my teaching colleagues, past and present, in the Stress Reduction Clinic and the Center for Mindfulness and, more recently, also to those teachers and researchers who are part of the CFM's global network of affiliate institutions. All have literally and metaphorically dedicated their lives and their passion to this work. At the time of the original book, those who had taught MBSR in the Stress Reduction Clinic for varying periods of time from 1979 to 2005 were Saki Santorelli, Melissa Blacker, Florence Meleo-Meyer, Elana Rosenbaum, Ferris Buck Urbanowski, Pamela Erdmann, Fernando de Torrijos, James Carmody, Danielle Levi Alvares, George Mumford, Diana Kamila, Peggy Roggenbuck-Gillespie, Debbie Beck, Zayda Vallejo, Barbara Stone, Trudy Goodman, Meg Chang, Larry Rosenberg, Kasey Carmichael, Franz Moekel, the late Ulli Kesper-Grossman, Maddy Klein, Ann Soulet, Joseph Koppel, the late Karen Ryder, Anna Klegon, Larry Pelz, Adi Bemak, Paul Galvin, and David Spound.

From 2005 to 2017, my admiration and gratitude go to the teachers at the Center for Mindfulness and its affiliate programs: Florence Meleo-Meyers, Lynn Koerbel, Elana Rosenbaum, Carolyn West, Bob Stahl, Meg Chang, Zayda Vallejo, Brenda Fingold, Dianne Horgan, Judson Brewer, Margaret Fletcher, Patti Holland, Rebecca Eldridge, Ted Meissner, Anne Twohig, Ana Arrabe, Beth Mulligan, Bonita Jones, Carola Garcia, Gustavo Diex, Beatriz Rodriguez, Melissa Tefft, Janet Solyntjes, Rob Smith, Jacob Piet, Claude Maskens, Charlotte Borch-Jacobsen, Christiane Wolf, Kate Mitcheom, Bob Linscott, Laurence Magro, Jim Colosi, Julie Nason, Lone Overby Fjorback, Dawn MacDonald, Leslie Smith Frank, Ruth Folchman, Colleen Camenisch, Robin Boudette, Eowyn Ahlstrom, Erin Woo, Franco Cuccio, Geneviève Hamelet, Gwenola Herbette, and Ruth Whitall. Florence Meleo-Meyer and Lynn Koerbel were outstanding leaders and nurturers of the global network of MBSR teachers at the CFM.

Profound appreciation to all those who contributed so critically in so many different ways to the administration of the MBSR Clinic and the Center for Mindfulness in Medicine, Health Care, and Society and to their various research and clinical endeavors from the very beginning: Norma Rosiello, Kathy Brady, Brian Tucker, Anne Skillings, Tim Light, Jean Baril, Leslie Lynch, Carol Lewis, Leigh Emery, Rafaela Morales, Roberta Lewis, Jen Gigliotti, Sylvia Ciario, Betty Flodin, Diane Spinney, Carol Hester, Carol Mento, Olivia Hobletzell, the late Narina Hendry, Marlene Samuelson, Janet Parks, Michael Bratt, Marc Cohen, and Ellen Wingard. For the period up to the spring of 2018, I extend my gratitude to Judson Brewer, Dianne Horgan, Florence Meleo-Meyer, Lynn Koerbel, Jean Baril, Jacqueline Clark, Tony Maciag, Ted Meissner, Jessica Novia, Maureen Titus, Beverly Walton, Ashley Gladden, Lynne Littizzio, Nicole Rocijewicz, and Jean Welker.

On the research side, robust appreciation for the contributions of the members of Judson Brewer's lab: Remko van Lutterveld, Prasanta Pal, Michael Datko, Andrea Ruf, Susan Druker, Ariel Beccia, Alexandra Roy, Hanif Benoit, Danny Theisen, and Carolyn Neal.

In the spring of 2018, the Center for Mindfulness underwent what I like to think of as a process of binary fission, with a number of people migrating to Brown University to establish a parallel and complementary mindfulness center and research program there under the aegis of the School of Public Health and the Medical School. I wish to express my gratitude to all involved in both institutions for what has been and what is yet to come in terms of clinical and professional training programs, research directions, and collaborative possibilities.

Finally, I would also like to express my gratitude and respect for the thousands of people everywhere around the world who work in or are researching mindfulness-based approaches in medicine, psychiatry, psychology, health care, education, the law, social justice, refugee healing in the face of trauma and sometimes genocide (as in South Darfur), childbirth and parenting, the workplace, government, prisons, and other facets of society, and who take care to honor the dharma in its universal depth and beauty in doing so. You know who you are, whether you are named here or not! And if you are not, it is only due to my own shortcomings and the limits of space. I want to explicitly honor the work of Paula Andrea Ramirez Diazgranados in Columbia and South Sudan; Hui Qi Tong in the U.S. and China; Kevin Fong, Roy Te Chung Chen, Tzungkuen Wen, Helen Ma, Jin Mei Hu, and Shih Shih Ming in China, Taiwan, and Hong Kong; Heyoung Ahn in Korea; Junko Bickel and Teruro Shiina in Japan; Leena Pennenen in Finland; Simon Whitesman and Linda Kantor in South Africa; Claude Maskens, Gwénola Herbette, Edel Max, Caroline Lesire, and Ilios Kotsou in Belgium; Jean-Gérard Bloch, Geneviève Hamelet, Marie-Ange Pratili, and Charlotte Borch-Jacobsen in France; Katherine Bonus, Trish Magyari, Erica Sibinga, David Kearney, Kurt Hoelting, Carolyn McManus, Mike Brumage, Maureen Strafford, Amy Gross, Rhonda Magee, George Mumford, Carl Fulwiler, Maria Kluge, Mick Krasner, Trish Luck, Bernice Todres, Ron Epstein, and Representative Tim Ryan in the U.S.: Paul Grossman, Maria Kluge, Sylvia Wiesman-Fiscalini, Linda Hehrhaupt, and Petra Meibert in Germany; Joke Hellemans, Johan Tinge, and Anna Speckens in Holland; Beatrice Heller and Regula Saner in Switzerland; Rebecca Crane, Willem Kuyken, John Teasdale, Mark Williams, Chris Cullen, Richard Burnett, Jamie Bristow, Trish Bartley, Stewart Mercer, Chris Ruane, Richard Layard, Guiaume Hung, and Ahn Nguyen in the UK; Zindel Segal and Norm Farb in Canada; Gabor Fasekas in Hungary; Macchi dela Vega in Argentina; Johan Bergstad, Anita Olsson, Angeli Holmstedt; Ola Schenström, and Camilla Sköld in Sweden; Andries Kroese in Norway; Jakob Piet and Lone Overby Fjorback in Denmark; and Franco Cuccio in Italy. May your work continue to reach those who are most in need of it, touching, clarifying, and nurturing what is deepest and best in us all, and thus contributing, in ways little and big to the healing and transformation that humanity so sorely longs for and aspires to.

RELATED READINGS

Mindfulness Meditation

Amero, B. *Small Boat, Great Mountain: Theravadan Reflections on the Great Natural Perfection*, Abhayagiri Monastic Foundation, Redwood Valley, CA, 2003.

Analayo, B. *Early Buddhist Meditation Studies*, Barre Center for Buddhist Studies, Barre, MA, 2017.

Analayo, B. *Mindfully Facing Disease and Death: Compassionate Advice from Early Buddhist Texts*, Windhorse, Cambridge, UK, 2016.

Analayo, B. *Sattipatthana Meditation: A Practice Guide*, Windhorse, Cambridge, UK, 2018.

Armstrong, G. *Emptiness: A Practical Guide for Meditators I*, Wisdom, Somerville, MA, 2017.

Beck, C. *Nothing Special: Living Zen*, HarperCollins, San Francisco, 1993.

Buswell, R. B., Jr. *Tracing Back the Radiance: Chinul's Korean Way of Zen*, Kuroda Institute, U of Hawaii Press, Honolulu, 1991.

Goldstein, J. *One Dharma: The Emerging Western Buddhism*, Harper, San Francisco, 2002.

Goldstein, J. and Kornfield, J. *Seeking the Heart of Wisdom: The Path of Insight Meditation*, Shambhala, Boston, 1987.

Gunaratana, H. *Mindfulness in Plain English*, Wisdom, Boston, 1996.

Hanh, T. N., *The Heart of the Buddha's Teachings*, Broadway, New York, 1998.

Hanh, T. N. *How to Love*, Parallax Press, Berkeley, 2015.

Hanh, T. N. *How to Sit*. Parallax Press, Berkeley, 2014.

Hanh, T. N., *The Miracle of Mindfulness*, Beacon, Boston, 1976.

Kapleau, P. *The Three Pillars of Zen: Teaching, Practice, and Enlightenment*, Random House, New York, 1965, 2000.

Krishnamurti, J. *This Light in Oneself: True Meditation*, Shambhala, Boston, 1999.

Levine, S. *A Gradual Awakening*, Anchor/Doubleday, Garden City, NY, 1979.

Rinpoche, M. *Joyful Wisdom*, Harmony Books, New York, 2010.

Ricard, M. *Happiness*, Little Brown, New York, 2007.

Ricard, M. *Why Meditate?* Hay House, New York, 2010.

Rosenberg, L. *Breath by Breath: The Liberating Practice of Insight Meditation*, Shambhala, Boston, 1998.

Rosenberg, L. *Living in the Light of Death: On the Art of Being Truly Alive*, Shambhala, Boston, 2000.

Rosenberg, L. *Three Steps to Awakening: A Practice for Bringing Mindfulness to Life*, Shambhala, Boston, 2013.

Salzberg, S. *Lovingkindness*, Shambhala, Boston, 1995.

Santorelli, S. *Heal Thy Self: Lessons on Mindfulness in Medicine*, Bell Tower, New York, 1999.

Soeng, M. *The Heart of the Universe: Exploring the Heart Sutra*, Wisdom, Somerville, MA, 2010.

Soeng, M. *Trust in Mind: The Rebellion of Chinese Zen*, Wisdom, Somerville, MA, 2004.

Sheng-Yen, C. *Hoofprints of the Ox: Principles of the Chan Buddhist Path*, Oxford University Press, New York, 2001.

Sumedo, A. *The Mind and the Way: Buddhist Reflections on Life*, Wisdom, Boston, 1995.

Suzuki, S. *Zen Mind, Beginner's Mind*, Weatherhill, New York, 1970.

Thera, N. *The Heart of Buddhist Meditation: The Buddha's Way of Mindfulness*, Red Wheel/Weiser, San Francisco, 1962, 2014.

Treleaven, D. *Trauma-Sensitive Mindfulness: Practices for Safe and Transformative Healing*, W.W. Norton, New York, 2018.

Urgyen, T. *Rainbow Painting*, Rangjung Yeshe, Boudhanath, Nepal, 1995.

MBSR

Brandsma, R. *The Mindfulness Teaching Guide: Essential Skills and Competencies for Teaching Mindfulness-Based Interventions*, New Harbinger, Oakland, CA, 2017.

Kabat-Zinn, J. *Full Catastrophe Living: Using the Wisdom of Your Body and Mind to Face Stress, Pain, and Illness*, revised and updated edition, Random House, New York, 2013.

Lehrhaupt, L. and Meibert, P. *Mindfulness-Based Stress Reduction: The MBSR Program for Enhancing Health and Vitality*, New World Library, Novato, CA, 2017.

Mulligan, B. A. *The Dharma of Modern Mindfulness: Discovering the Buddhist Teachings at the Heart of Mindfulness-Based Stress Reduction*, New Harbinger, Oakland, CA, 2017.

Rosenbaum, E. *The Heart of Mindfulness-Based Stress Reduction: An MBSR Guide for Clinicians and Clients*, Pesi Publishing, Eau Claire, WI, 2017.

Santorelli, S. *Heal Thy Self: Lessons on Mindfulness in Medicine*, Bell Tower, New York, 1999.

Stahl, B., and Goldstein, E. *A Mindfulness-Based Stress Reduction Workbook*, New Harbinger, Oakland, CA, 2010.

Stahl, B., Meleo-Meyer, F, and Koerbel, L. *A Mindfulness-Based Stress Reduction Workbook for Anxiety*, New Harbinger, Oakland, CA, 2014.

Applications of Mindfulness and Other Books on Meditation

Baer, R.A. (ed.). *Mindfulness-Based Treatment Approaches: Clinician's Guide to Evidence Base and Applications*, Academic Press, Waltham, MA, 2014.

Bennett-Goleman, T. *Emotional Alchemy: How the Mind Can Heal the Heart*, Harmony, New York, 2001.

Bögels, S. and Restifo, K. *Mindful Parenting: A Guide for Mental Health Practitioners*, Springer, New York, 2014.

Brantley, J. *Calming Your Anxious Mind: How Mindfulness and Compassion Can Free You from Anxiety, Fear, and Panic*, New Harbinger, Oakland, CA, 2003.

Crane, R. *Mindfulness-Based Cognitive Therapy*, Routledge, New York, 2017.

Epstein, M. *Thoughts Without a Thinker*, Basic Books, New York, 1995.

Ergas, O. *Reconstructing "Education" Through Mindful Attention: Positioning the Mind at the Center of Curriculum and Pedagogy*, Palgrave Macmillan, London, UK, 2017.

Gazzaley, A. and Rosen, L. D. *The Distracted Mind: Ancient Brains in a High-Tech World*, MIT Press, Cambridge, MA, 2016.

Germer, C. K. and Siegel, R. D. (eds.). *Wisdom and Compassion in Psychotherapy: Deepeing Mindfulness in Clinical Practice*, Guilford, New York, 2012.

Germer, C. K., Siegel, R. D., and Fulton, P. R. (eds.). *Mindfulness and Psychotherapy*, Guilford, New York, 2005.

Goleman, D. *Destructive Emotions: How We Can Heal Them*, Bantam, New York, 2003.

Hasenkamp, W. *The Monastery and the Microscope: Conversations with the Dalai Lama on Mind, Mindfulness, and the Nature of Reality*, Yale, New Haven, 2017.

Himmelstein, S. and Stephen, S. *Mindfulness-Based Substance Abuse Treatment for Adolescents—A 12 Session Curriculum*, Routledge, New York, 2016.

Kabat-Zinn, J. *Mindfulness for Beginners: Reclaiming the Present Moment—and Your Life*, Sounds True, Boulder, CO, 2012.

Kabat-Zinn, J. *Wherever You Go, There You Are: Mindfulness Meditation in Every day Life*, Hachette, 1994, 2005.

Kabat-Zinn, J. and Davidson, R. J. *The Mind's Own Physician: A Scientific Dialogue with the Dalai Lama on the Healing Power of Meditation*, New Harbinger, Oakland, CA, 2011.

Kabat-Zinn, M. and Kabat-Zinn, J. *Everyday Blessings: The Inner Work of Mindful Parenting*, Hachette, New York, 1997, Revised 2014.

King, R. *Mindful of Race: Transforming Racism from the Inside Out.* Sounds True, Boulder, CO, 2018.

Martins, C. *Mindfulness-Based Interventions for Older Adults: Evidence for Practice,* Jessica Langley, Philadelphia, PA, 2014.

Mason-John, V. and Groves, P. Eight-Step Recovery: *Using the Buddha's Teachings to Overcome Addiction,* Windhorse, Cambridge, UK, 2018.

McBee, L. Mindfulness-Based Elder Care: *A CAM Model for Frail Elders and Their Caregivers,* Springer, New York, 2008.

McManus, C. A. *Group Wellness Programs for Chronic Pain and Disease Management,* Butterworth-Heinemann, St. Louis, MO, 2003.

Miller, L. D. *Effortless Mindfulness: Genuine Mental Health Through Awakened Presence,* Routledge, New York, 2014.

Pollak, S. M., Pedulla, T., and Siegel, R. D. *Sitting Together: Essential Skills for Mindfulness-Based Psychotherapy,* Guilford, New York, 2014.

Rossy, L. *The Mindfulness-Based Eating Solution: Proven Strategies to End Overeating, Satisfy Your Hunger, and Savor Your Life,* New Harbinger, Oakland, CA, 2016.

Segal, Z. V., Williams, J.M.G., and Teasdale, J. D. *Mindfulness-Based Cognitive Therapy for Depression: A New Approach to Preventing Relapse,* Guilford, NY, 2002.

Silverton, S. *The Mindfulness Breakthrough: The Revolutionary Approach to Dealing with Stress, Anxiety, and Depression,* Watkins, London, UK, 2012.

Smalley, S. L. and Winston, D. *Fully Present: The Science, Art, and Practice of Mindfulness,* DaCapo, Philadelphia, PA, 2010.

Tolle, E. *The Power of Now,* New World Library, Novato, CA, 1999.

Vo, D. X. *The Mindful Teen: Powerful Skills to Help You Handle Stress One Moment at a Time,* New Harbinger, Oakland, Ca., 2015.

Wallace, B. A. *Tibetan Buddhism from the Ground Up,* Wisdom, Somerville, MA, 1993.

Williams, J.M.G., Teasdale, J. D., Segal, Z. V., and Kabat-Zinn, J. *The Mindful Way Through Depression: Freeing Yourself from Chronic Unhappiness,* Guilford, NY, 2007

Williams, M., Fennell, M., Barnhofeer, T., Crane, R., and Silverton, S. *Mindfulness and the Transformation of Despair: Working with People at Risk of Suicide,* Guilford, New York, 2015.

Williams, M. and Kabat-Zinn, J. (eds.). *Mindfulness: Diverse Perspectives on Its Meaning, Origins, and Applications,* Routledge, Abingdon, UK, 2013.

Wright, R. *Why Buddhism Is True: The Science and Philosophy of Meditation and Enlightenment,* Simon & Schuster, 2018.

Yang, L. *Awakening Together: The Spiritual Practice of Inclusivity and Community,* Wisdom, Somerville, MA, 2017.

Other Applications of Mindfulness

Bardacke, N. *Mindful Birthing: Training the Mind, Body, and Heart for Childbirth and Beyond*, HarperCollins, New York, 2012.

Bartley, T. *Mindfulness-Based Cognitive Therapy for Cancer*, Wiley-Blackwell, West Sussex, UK, 2012.

Bartley, T. *Mindfulness: A Kindly Approach to Cancer*, Wiley-Blackwell, West Sussex, UK, 2016.

Bays, J. C. *Mindful Eating: A Guide to Rediscovering a Healthy and Joyful Relationship with Food*, Shambhala, Boston, 2009, 2017.

Bays, J. C. *Mindfulness on the Go: Simple Meditation Practices You Can Do Anywhere*, Shambhala, Boston, 2014.

Biegel, G. *The Stress-Reduction Workbook for Teens: Mindfulness Skills to Help You Deal with Stress*, New Harbinger, Oakland, CA 2017.

Brown, K. W., Creswell, J. D., and Ryan, R.M. (eds.). *Handbook of Mindfulness: Theory, Research, and Practice*, Guilford, New York, 2015.

Carlson, L., and Speca, M. *Mindfulness-Based Cancer Recovery: A Step-by-Step MBSR Approach to Help You Cope with Treatment and Reclaim Your Life*, New Harbinger, Oakland, CA, 2010.

Cullen, M., and Pons, G. B. *The Mindfulness-Based Emotional Balance Workbook: An Eight-Week Program for Improved Emotion Regulation and Resilience*, New Harbinger, Oakland, CA, 2015.

Germer, C. *The Mindful Path to Self-Compassion*, Guilford, New York, 2009.

Greenland, S. K. *The Mindful Child*, Free Press, New York, 2010.

Greenland, S. K. *Mindful Games: Sharing Mindfulness and Meditation with Children, Teens, and Families*, Shambhala, Boulder, CO, 2016.

Gunaratana, B. H. *Mindfulness in Plain English*, Wisdom, Somerville, MA, 2002.

Jennings, P. *Mindfulness for Teachers: Simple Skills for Peace and Productivity in the Classroom*, W.W. Norton, New York, 2015.

McCown, D., Reibel, D., and Micozzi, M. S. (eds.). *Resources for Teaching Mindfulness: An International Handbook*, Springer, New York, 2016.

McCown, D., Reibel, D., and Micozzi, M. S. (eds.). *Teaching Mindfulness: A Practical Guide for Clinicians and Educators*, Springer, New York, 2010.

Mumford, G. *The Mindful Athlete: Secrets to Pure Performance*, Parallax Press, Berkeley, 2015.

Penman, D. *The Art of Breathing*, Conari, Newburyport, MA, 2018.

Rechtschaffen, D. *The Mindful Education Workbook: Lessons for Teaching Mindfulness to Students*, W.W. Norton, New York, 2016.

Rechtschaffen, D. *The Way of Mindful Education: Cultivating Wellbeing in Teachers and Students*, W.W. Norton, New York, 2014.

Rosenbaum, E. *Being Well (Even When You're Sick): Mindfulness Practices for People with Cancer and Other Serious Illnesses*, Shambala, Boston, 2012.

Rosenbaum, E. *Here for Now: Living Well with Cancer Through Mindfulness,* Satya House, Hardwick, MA, 2005.

Williams, A. K., Owens, R., and Syedullah, J. *Radical Dharma: Talking Race, Love, and Liberation,* North Atlantic Books, Berkeley, 2016.

Williams, M., and Penman, D. *Mindfulness: An Eight-Week Plan for Finding Peace in a Frantic World,* Rodale, 2012.

Yoga and Stretching

Boccio, F. J. *Mindfulness Yoga,* Wisdom, Boston, 2004.

Christensen, A. and Rankin, D. *Easy Does It Yoga: Yoga for Older People,* Harper & Row, New York, 1979.

Iyengar, B.K.S. *Light on Yoga,* revised edition, Schocken, New York, 1977.

Kraftsow, G. *Yoga for Wellness,* Penguin/Arkana, New York, 1999.

Meyers, E. *Yoga and You,* Random House Canada, Toronto, 1996.

Healing

Doidge, N. *The Brain's Way of Healing: Remarkable Discoveries and Recoveries from the Frontiers of Neuroplasticity,* Penguin Random House, 2016.

Goleman, D. *Healing Emotions: Conversations with the Dalai Lama on Mindfulness, Emotions, and Health,* Shambhala, Boston, 1997.

Halpern, S. *The Etiquette of Illness: What to Say When You Can't Find the Words,* Bloomsbury, New York, 2004.

Lazare, A. *On Apology,* Oxford, New York, 2004.

Lerner, M. *Choices in Healing: Integrating the Best of Conventional and Complementary Approaches to Cancer,* MIT Press, Cambridge, MA, 1994.

Meili, T. *I Am the Central Park Jogger,* Scribner, New York, 2003.

Moyers, B. *Healing and the Mind,* Doubleday, New York, 1993.

Ornish, D. *Love and Survival: The Scientific Basis for the Healing Power of Intimacy,* HaperCollins, New York, 1998.

Remen, R. *Kitchen Table Wisdom: Stories that Heal,* Riverhead, New York, 1997.

Siegel, D. *The Mindful Brain: Reflection and Attunement in the Cultivation of Well-Being,* W.W. Norton, New York, 2007.

Simmons, P. *Learning to Fall: The Blessings of an Imperfect Life,* Bantam, New York, 2002.

Tarrant, J. *The Light Inside the Dark: Zen, Soul, and the Spiritual Life,* HarperCollins, New York, 1998.

Tenzin Gyatso (the 14th Dalai Lama). *The Compassionate Life,* Wisdom, Boston, 2003.

Van der Kolk, B. *The Body Keeps the Score: Brain, Mind, and Body in the Healing of Trauma,* Penguin Random House, New York, 2014.

Poetry

Bly, R. *The Soul Is Here for Its Own Joy,* Ecco, Hopewell, NJ, 1995.

Eliot, T. S. *Four Quartets,* Harcourt Brace, New York, 1943, 1977.

Lao-Tzu, *Tao Te Ching* (Stephen Mitchell, transl.), HarperCollins, New York, 1988.

Mitchell, S. *The Enlightened Heart,* Harper & Row, New York, 1989.

Oliver, M. *New and Selected Poems,* Beacon, Boston, 1992.

Tanahashi, K., and Levitt, P. *The Complete Cold Mountain: Poems of the Legendary Hermit Hanshan.* Shambhala, Boulder, CO, 2018.

Whyte, D. *The Heart Aroused: Poetry and the Preservation of the Soul in Corporate America,* Doubleday, New York, 1994.

Other Books of Interest, some Mentioned in the Text

Abram, D. *The Spell of the Sensuous,* Vintage, New York, 1996.

Ackerman, D. *A Natural History of the Senses,* Vintage, New York, 1990.

Bohm, D. *Wholeness and the Implicate Order,* Routledge and Kegan Paul, London, 1980.

Bryson, B. *A Short History of Nearly Everything,* Broadway, New York, 2003.

Davidson, R. J., and Begley, S. *The Emotional Life of Your Brain,* Hudson St. Press, New York, 2012.

Glassman, B. *Bearing Witness: A Zen Master's Lessons in Making Peace,* Bell Tower, New York, 1998.

Greene, B. *The Elegant Universe,* Norton, New York, 1999.

Harari, Y. N. *Sapiens: A Brief History of Humankind,* HarperCollins, New York, 2015.

Hillman, J. *The Soul's Code: In Search of Character and Calling,* Random House, New York, 1996.

Karr-Morse, R., and Wiley, M. S. *Ghosts from the Nursery: Tracing the Roots of Violence,* Atlantic Monthly Press, New York, 1997.

Katie, B., and Mitchell, S. *A Mind at Home with Itself,* HarperCollins, New York, 2017.

Kazanjian, V. H., and Laurence, P. L. (eds.). *Education as Transformation,* Peter Lang, New York, 2000.

Kurzweil, R. *The Age of Spiritual Machines,* Viking, New York, 1999.

Luke, H. *Old Age: Journey into Simplicity,* Parabola, New York, 1987.

Montague, A. *Touching: The Human Significance of the Skin,* Harper & Row, New York, 1978.

Palmer, P. *The Courage to Teach: Exploring the Inner Landscape of a Teacher's Life,* Jossey-Bass, San Francisco, 1998.

Pinker, S. *The Better Angles of Our Nature: Why Violence Has Declined*, Penguin Random House, New York, 2012.

Pinker, S. *Enlightenment Now: The Case for Reason, Science, Humanism, and Progress*, Viking, New York, 2018.

Pinker, S. *How the Mind Works*, Norton, New York, 1997.

Ravel, J.-F. and Ricard, M. *The Monk and the Philosopher: A Father and Son Discuss the Meaning of Life*, Schocken, New York, 1998.

Ricard, M. *Altruism: The Power of Compassion to Change Yourself and the World*, Little Brown, New York, 2013.

Ryan, T. *A Mindful Nation: How a Simple Practice Can Help Us Reduce Stress, Improve Performance, and Recapture the American Spirit*, Hay House, New York, 2012.

Sachs, J. D. *The Price of Civilization: Reawakening American Virtue and Prosperity*, Random House, New York, 2011.

Sachs, O. *The Man Who Mistook His Wife for a Hat*, Touchstone, New York, 1970.

Sachs, O. *The River of Consciousness*, Knopf, New York, 2017.

Sapolsky, R. *Behave: The Biology of Humans at Our Best and Worst*, Penguin Random House, New York, 2017.

Scarry, E. *Dreaming by the Book*, Farrar, Straus & Giroux, New York, 1999.

Schwartz, J. M. and Begley, S. *The Mind and the Brain: Neuroplasticity and the Power of Mental Force*, HarperCollins, New York, 2002.

Singh, S. *Fermat's Enigma*, Anchor, New York, 1997.

Tanahashi, K. *The Heart Sutra: A Comprehensive Guide to the Classic of Mahayana Buddhism*, Shambhala, Boulder, CO, 2016.

Tegmark, M. *Life 3.0: Being Human in the Age of Artificial Intelligence*, Knopf, New York, 2017.

Tegmark, M. *The Mathematical Universe: My Quest for the Ultimate Nature of Reality*, Knopf, New York, 2014.

Varela, F. J., Thompson, E., and Rosch, E. *The Embodied Mind: Cognitive Science and Human Experience*, revised edition, MIT Press, Cambridge, MA, 2017.

Websites

www.umassmed.edu/cfm	Website of the Center for Mindfulness, UMass Medical School
www.mindandlife.org	Website of the Mind and Life Institute
www.dharma.org	Vipassana retreat centers and schedules

INDEX

ABOUT THE AUTHOR

JON KABAT-ZINN, Ph.D., is the founder of MBSR (mindfulness-based stress reduction) and the Stress Reduction Clinic (1979) and of the Center for Mindfulness in Medicine, Health Care, and Society (1995) at the University of Massachusetts Medical School. He is also professor of Medicine emeritus. He leads workshops and retreats on mindfulness for health professionals, the tech and business communities, and for lay audiences worldwide. He is a strong proponent of social justice and economic justice. He is the author or coauthor of fourteen books, including the bestselling *Wherever You Go, There You Are* and *Full Catastrophe Living*. With his wife Myla Kabat-Zinn, he published a book on mindful parenting, *Everyday Blessings*. He has been featured in numerous documentaries for television around the world, including the PBS Special *Healing and the Mind* with Bill Moyers, *Oprah*, and CBS's *60 Minutes* with Anderson Cooper. He lives in Massachusetts. His work has contributed to a growing movement of mindfulness into mainstream institutions such as medicine, psychology, health care, neuroscience, schools, higher education, business, social justice, criminal justice, prisons, the law, technology, government, and professional sports. Hospitals and medical centers around the world now offer clinical programs based on training in mindfulness and MBSR.

Continue the journey and get the full set of Jon Kabat-Zinn's four small-but-mighty guides to mindfulness and meditation, as well as his bestselling classic *Wherever You Go, There You Are*.

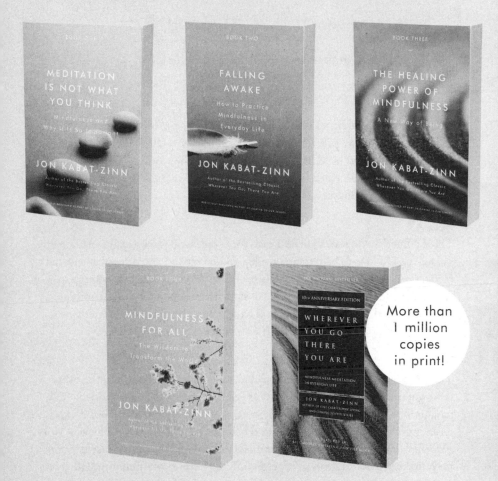

More than 1 million copies in print!

JON KABAT-ZINN, PhD, is the founder of Mindfulness-Based Stress Reduction (MBSR) and of the Center for Mindfulness in Medicine, Health Care and Society at the University of Massachusetts, where he is Professor of Medicine emeritus. He is the author of numerous bestselling books about mindfulness and meditation. For more information, visit www.jonkabat-zinn.com.

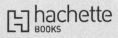 hachette BOOKS

Guided Mindfulness Meditation Practices with Jon Kabat-Zinn

Obtainable as apps, downloads, or CDs
(see below for links)

Series 1

These guided meditations (the body scan and sitting meditation) and guided mindful yoga practices 1 and 2 form the foundational practices of MBSR and are used in MBSR programs around the world. These practices and their use are described in detail in *Full Catastrophe Living*. Each meditation is 45 minutes in length.

Series 2

These guided meditations are designed for people who want a range of shorter guided meditations to help them develop and/or expand and deepen a personal meditation practice based on mindfulness. The series includes the mountain and lake meditations (each 20 minutes) as well as a range of other 10-minute, 20-minute, and 30-minute sitting and lying down practices. This series was originally developed to accompany *Wherever You Go, There You Are*.

Series 3

These guided meditations are designed to accompany this book and the other three volumes based on *Coming to Our Senses*. Series 3 includes guided meditations on the breath and body sensations (breathscape and bodyscape), on sounds (soundscape), thoughts and emotions (mindscape), choiceless awareness (nowscape), and lovingkindness (heartscape), as well as instructions for lying down meditation (corpse pose/dying before you die), mindful walking, and cultivating mindfulness in everyday life (lifescape).

For iPhone and Android apps: www.mindfulnessapps.com

For digital downloads: www.betterlisten.com/pages/jonkabatzinnseries123

For CD sets: www.soundstrue.com/jon-kabat-zinn